Rheumatoid Diseases *CURED* at Last

by
Anthony di Fabio

D0032155

A Publication of *The Rheumatoid Disease Foundation*

A Publication of *The Rheumatoid Disease Foundation*

Publisher certifies that this is an independent news report made as accurately as possible, and further certifies that no drug company, medical doctor, or medically related institution has any financial interest in the sale and proceeds of this publication or the medicines recommended. Publisher further advises that all treatment should be through a licensed physician, and that we cannot be responsible for mal-application or mis-application or inappropriate treatment of any kind. Voluntary contributions to the tax-exempt, charitable The Roger Wyburn-Mason and Jack M. Blount Foundation for Eradication of Rheumatoid Disease, Inc. *(The Rheumatoid Disease Foundation), P.O. Box 17405, Washington, D.C. 20041, will be used for the purpose of furthering research and in communicating discoveries.*

Library of Congress Cataloging Number 82-73215

ISBN 0-931150-12-4 $9.95 plus $1.00 postage and handling or free premium for $15.00 Donation.

Published by *The Rheumatoid Disease Foundation*
Rt. 4, Box 137, Franklin, TN 37064
(615) 646-1030
Typesetting and Layout by *AC Projects, Inc.*
Franklin, TN 37064
Printed in Washington, DC, USA

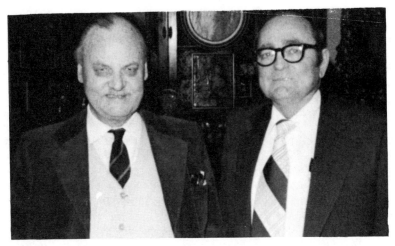

Roger Wyburn-Mason, M.D., Ph.D. and Jack M. Blount, Jr., M.D.

Dedication and Acknowledgement

This book is dedicated to two brilliant and brave men, Professor Roger Wyburn-Mason, who one day should receive the Nobel Prize in Medicine, and Dr. Jack M. Blount, who should at least receive the Congressional Medal of Honor for bravery in the face of hostile forces; with special mention also for Dr. Robert Bingham whose open-mindedness and foresight brought Professor Roger Wyburn-Mason's work overseas, John R.A. Simoons, Ph.D., for persistence in bringing this work to attention of academia and drug manufacturers, Dr. Archimedes A. Concon, for vision in applications, and Dr. Eugene S. Wolcott who knows why; and an additional personal thanks to L. Ron Hubbard and John W. Campbell, Jr. for providing the author with vision on the coin's other side.

Physicians and Scientists Advisory Committee of *The Roger Wyburn-Mason and Jack M. Blount Foundation for Eradication of Rheumatoid Disease* (*The Rheumatoid Disease Foundation*), have been particularly helpful in creating new medical protocol and in disseminating rheumatoid disease information, for which a deep, heartfelt thanks —.

This book is a report of the life-time work of Professor Roger Wyburn-Mason, who had for more than twenty-six years researched the roles of pathogenic protozoa in human diseases as a protozoologist, pharmacologist and rheumatologist.

In collaboration with his wife, and over twelve years, he wrote a monumental work, which may revolutionize the diagnosis and treatment of many chronic and dangerous illnesses. The work is titled *The Causation of Rheumatoid Disease and Many Human Cancers — A New Concept in Medicine*[1].

The material that follows in this book for the most part is taken from

i

Professor Roger Wyburn-Mason's primary book and/or his *Addenda*, (*The Causation of Rheumatoid Disease and Many Human Cancers — A New Concept in Medicine — A Pre'cis and Addenda, Including the Nature of Multiple Sclerosis*) with his permission. The Memoriam below is from the rear cover of Roger's *Addenda*, his last book to be published.

We also wish to acknowledge and to share with the reader our appreciation for the more than generous cooperation of the many people who helped us. They are: Branch Owen Adkerson (Franklin, TN, USA), Stan J. Bardo (Pietermaritzburg, Republic of South Africa), Frederick H. Binford (Nashville, TN, USA), Carol Blount (Philadelphia, MS, USA), William E. Catterall (Tucson, AZ, USA), Warren B. Causey (San Antonio, TX, USA), E. Harrison Clark (Alexandria, VA, USA), Terry Crommelin (Perth, Western Australia), Robert Edmonds (Hollywood, CA, USA), George Hay (London, England), Kay Hitchen (Southampton, Hampshire, England), Carl Hosch, Jr. (Atlanta, GA, USA), Bob Kemp (Beebe, AR, USA), John Kern, (Brentwood, TN, USA), Jean Lancaster (Philadelphia, MS, USA), Gus and Patty J. Prosch, Jr. (Birmingham, AL, USA), Paul K. Pybus (Pietermaritzburg, South Africa) Carl J. Reich (Calgary, Alberta, Canada), Larry L. Roberts (Nashville, TN, USA), Don and Nancy Vansant (Nashville, TN, USA), Joan Wyburn-Mason (London, England), Vaughn Young (Hollywood, CA, USA), and many others, some of whom prefer anonymity.

In Memoriam
Roger Wyburn-Mason   Oct. 2, 1911 — June 16, 1983

When I was at last cured of the dreaded, crippling rheumatoid arthritis, I never dreamed of embarking on a world-wide challenge to professional rheumatologists, the gigantic and ineffective Arthritis Foundation, and the American petrochemical industry that siphons $15,000,000,000 a year in the United States of America from the sick and the lonely, chiefly for aspirin substitutes that simply treat symptoms, and not causes.

Somehow the Good Lord has seen fit to successfully guide my path — along with other determined, sincere people — to bring the good message to all: there is a cure! it is simple! it is cheap! it is available everywhere!

My book *Rheumatoid Diseases Cured at Last* (1982) was monitored by Professor Roger Wyburn-Mason, and based on his original work, *The Causation of Rheumatoid Disease and Many Human Cancers* (1978). My book was designed for the ailing to find hope, to convince them, to be carried to their family physician for further interpretation where they would be treated.

My small book also launched *The Roger Wyburn-Mason & Jack M. Blount Foundation for Eradication of Rheumatoid Disease (The Rheumatoid Disease*

Foundation), which is now successfully off and running, millions of messages spreading the word. Many fine humanity-conscious physicians and non-physicians are now members, and working toward common goals set by Professor Roger Wyburn-Mason. Some six weeks ago I wrote to Roger, asking that he please include a summary of his professional life and writings. I argued that while his work ought to stand on its own two feet, professional humans, like other humans, simply were more impressed with the number of "brownie points" and "merit badges" than with whether or not the work was "scientifically valid" — not meaning, of course, to disparage either the Boy or Girl Scouts, (I was an active Boy Scout) but rather to emphasize the sad state in which the so-called professional scientific community finds itself — where "altitude" and "prestige" is of more consequence than scientific validity.

Reluctantly, Professor Roger Wyburn-Mason sent this, his last letter before the Good Lord called him on June 16, 1983.

"I was born in Monmouthsire, England. On my mother's side I am a descendent of Bishop Stephen Gardiner, who was Lord Chancellor of England, that is the most powerful person in the country after the Monarch in the reign of King Henry VIII, King Edward VI, Queen Mary the first and Queen Elizabeth the first. He conducted the marriage of King Philip II of Spain to Queen Mary the first of England in Winchester Cathederal, where he is buried in a magnificent tomb. My mother's cousin was the former Prime Minister of New Zealand, Mr. Nash. My godfathers were the greatest English Composer, Dr. Ralph Vaughan Williams of Cambridge University and now buried in Westminster Abbey, and the historian H.A.L. Fisher, the head of New College Oxford, both of whom held the decoration of Order of Merit (O.M.), the highest honour that can be bestowed by the Monarch.

"I attended a public school (a public school in England is the opposite of one in the United States, being privately as opposed to state owned and includes such distinguished Institutions as Eton, Harrow and Winchester Colleges). At the end of school years I took the necessary final examinations and gained the top marks in the whole of Great Britain and was awarded a State Scholarship and an Open Scholarship to Christ's College, Cambridge (founded in 1405 A.D.), where the poet John Milton and the great scientist Charles Darwin were also students. Here I occupied the same rooms as those of Darwin himself.

"At Cambridge I obtained double first class honours in the final examinations for the B.A. (Bachelor of Arts) degree. I also represented my University at Rugby football and Athletics. At the end of my period as an Undergraduate I remained in Cambridge as a Bachelor Fellow of the College and did research in pathology and particularly protozoology. I afterwards was awarded the degree of M.A. (Master of Arts) a higher degree and the only University scholarship awarded to graduates completing their clinical studies at a London Hospital where I finally obtained my M.B. (Bachelor of Medicine) and B. Chir. (Bachelor of Chirurgerie). I afterwards held the posts of Registrar (the equivalent of Instructor in America) in the foremost hospitals in London, namely the Middlesex Hospital, the Brompton Hospital for Chest Diseases, the National Heart Hospital, the National Hospital for Nervous Diseases and the Royal Marsden Hospital for Cancer. While at the Middlesex Hospital I took part in the first Clinical Trials of the first sulphonamide Antibiotics. While working at the National Hospital for Nervous Diseases I wrote my thesis for the M.D. (Cambridge Degree — This is a higher degree unlike it is in the United States and other countries). I also sat for M.R.C.P. (Member of the Royal College of Physicians) examination in which I obtained the top marks of all the candidates. My M.D. thesis was entitled "The vascular tumours and abnormalities of the spinal cord and its membranes" and received with acclaim as it was the first description of these matters. It was published as a monograph and has remained the standard work on this subject. While working at the National Hospital for Nervous Diseases I published a number of papers in Medical Journals and two of these described new diseases which have since been named after me and I am the only *living* doctor who has such a distinction. One of these conditions describes the presentation of cancer as a peripheral neuropathy, that is a disturbance of the nerves of the limbs before any other evidence of cancer is present. The other describes a congenital blood vessel disease of the skin of the forehead, the fundus of the eye, the optic nerve and the brain.

"I later was elected Research Fellow at the Royal Marsden Hospital for research into cancer and later Research Fellow at the Royal College of Surgeons of England, where I continued my research into the nature of cancer and first isolated from all human malignant tumours and from cases of rheumatoid arthritis an hitherto unknown, very small free-living amoeba. For this I received the Ph.D. degree.

"While working at the Royal Marsden Hospital I discovered that human tissues affected by herpes zoster (shingles) and by herpes simplex (cold sores) which are both due to virus infections, were liable to develop cancer of the skin at a later date. This was the first description of human cancer caused by a virus and it resulted in my invitation by the late Professor Duran-Reynals, who was working at Yale University on the viral cause of human cancer, to Yale to work with him as his assistant where I continued after his death. I later transferred to the Mayo Clinic and worked with the late Dr. J.W. Kernohan, the neuropathologist.

"I became convinced that while viruses cause cancer in animals, they rarely do so in man. During these years I published many papers and monographs (books) on my researches, and as a result of these I was awarded the degree of Doctor of Science of Cambridge University (a rare honour) and elected a Fellow of my old College.

"After twenty years work on the new organism which I had discovered I was able to show that this was the cause of rheumatoid arthritis. Furthermore, infection with species of this organism in susceptible subjects seemed to be the cause of a large proportion of cases of human cancer, which can be prevented by taking appropriate substances which kill the organism. This work has all been described in a book entitled *The causation of rheumatoid disease and many human cancers — A new concept in Medicine*, and it has caused worldwide interest.

"After a time it became necessary for me to return to England where I continued my work in the laboratories and wards of the National Health Service.

"Among my publications are the following —

Books

The vascular tumours and abnormalities of the spinal cord and its membranes. Henry Kimpton, London, 1943.
Trophic nerves. Henry Kimpton, London, 1950.
Reticulo-endothelial system in growth and tumour formation. Henry Kimpton, London, 1958.

A new protozoon, its relation to malignant and other diseases. Henry Kimpton, London, 1964.

The causation of rheumatoid disease and many human cancers — a New concept in Medicine. Iji Publishing Co. Tokyo, Japan, 1978.

A précis and addendum to the above. AC Publishing Co., Rt. 4, Box 137, Franklin, TN 37064, 1983.

Some Papers

"On some anomalous forms of amaurotic idiocy and their bearing on the relationship of various types". *Brit. Journ. Ophthalmol.*, April/May 1943, p. 145-187.

"Arterio-venous aneurysm of midbrain and retina, facial naevi and mental changes". *Brain*, 1943, 66, 163-203. (This is known as *Wyburn-Mason Syndrome I*).

"On some pressure effects associated with cervical and the rudimentary and 'normal' first ribs and the factors entering into their causation". *Brain*, 1944, 67, 141-177.

"A new conception of angina pectoris". *Brit. Med. J.*, 1948, i, 972.

"Bronchial carcinoma presenting as polyneuritis". (*Wyburn-Mason's Syndrome II*). *Lancet*, 1948, i, 203.

"The significance of the reference of anginal pain to the right or left side of the body". *Amer. Heart J., 1950, 39, 325-335.*

"The nature of tic doulourux". *Brit. Med. J.*, 1953, iii, 119.

"Costo-clavicular compression of the subclavian vein and its significance in relation to post operative oedema in carcinoma of the breast". *Brit. Med. J.*, 1953, iv, 1198-1200.

"Nature of Bell's palsy". *Brit. Med. J.*, 1954, iii, 679-681.

"Malignant change arising in tissues affected by herpes simplex". *Brit. Med. J.*, 1955, iv, 1106-1109.

"Malignant change following herpes simplex". *Brit. Med. J.*, 1957, ii, 615-161.

"Visceral lesions in herpes zoster". *Brit. Med. J.*, 1957, i, 678-681.

These last three articles are the first reports of a viral cause of human cancer.

"Association of gastroduodenal lesions with Me'nie're's syndrome". *Brit. Med. J.*, 1959, i, 78-83.

"Clotrimazole and rheumatoid arthritis". *Lancet*, 1976, i. 489.

"The free-living amoebic causation of rheumatoid and auto-immune diseases". *International Medicine*, 1979, 1, 20-25.

"New views on the aetiology of rheumatoid arthritis". *British Medicine*, August 21st, p. 12-14.

"The Naegerial causation of rheumatoid disease and many human cancers — A new concept in medicine". *Medical Hypotheses*, 1979, 5, 1237-1249.

"SLE and lymphoma". *Lancet*, January 20th, 1979.

"ROGER WYBURN-MASON   June 10th, 1983"

Professor Roger Wyburn-Mason solved the riddle of one of man's oldest curses, and in so doing, discovered a vast panorama of formerly, and so-called, incurable diseases. He strived with every ounce of his great, God-given intellect to bring to all humanity his discoveries. We prayed to be there when he walked across the stage to receive his Nobel Prize, and other prizes that were his due — but God, in his great wisdom, decided otherwise for us, and we must accept.

To the famous names of Semmelweis, Jenner, Koch, Harvey, Ross, Lister, Pasteur, Ehrlich, Sister Kenny, and Roentgen add Wyburn-Mason — a most brilliant, brave, humanity-loving man who pursued evil forces causing them to acknowledge that humanity need not always feel pain, suffering, depression, disillusionment —.

The simple antiamoebic cures developed by Professor Roger Wyburn-Mason, M.D., Jack M. Blount, M.D., and Robert Bingham, M.D. are described herein; and corroboratory case histories are also included.

In Memoriam

Mrs. Joan Wyburn-Mason, the beautiful lady who patiently supported and worked with Roger Wyburn-Mason through his many brilliant medical discoveries, died March 1, 1985.

Her last work, in support of her former husband, is entitled *Dedication, Love and Humour*, a brief biography of their life together, as told through Joan's loving eyes.

This well-written manuscript will be published by *The Rheumatoid Disease Foundation*.

---

[1] Professor Roger Wyburn-Mason's book *The Causation of Rheumatoid Disease and Many Human Cancers*, was originally only available in Japan at $125 each. Limited numbers have been placed in various hospital and university medical libraries, at Dr. Jack M. Blount's expense. The book will be republished by *The Rheumatoid Disease Foundation* in the future. During the interim, write to *The Foundation* for information on obtaining loan copies. The *Addenda* is available through *The Rheumatoid Disease Foundation* [$7.50 plus $1.00 postage].

Table of Contents

Photographs and Drawings

Preface

Cooperating physicians have successfully treated tens of thousands of patients afflicted with so-called incurable rheumatoid diseases using a low-cost, simple medical procedure.

The American Medical Association estimates some *13 million Americans seek relief from rheumatoid arthritis.* Three million are restricted in their daily activities. Seven hundred thousand cannot do useful work, keep house, attend school or enjoy recreational activities.

The April 24, 1983 Arthritis Foundation National Telethon (out of Nashville, TN) stated that one out of every three people will suffer from some form of arthritis, that one person contracts the disease every 33 seconds.

Dr. Carolyne K. Davis[1] of the U.S. Department of Health and Human Services stated that the U.S. Medicare program costs the U.S. Government about one billion dollars annually for rheumatoid diseases; and that probably an equal annual amount is spent through State Medicaid programs, totalling U.S. Citizens about two billion dollars per year for treatment and care of those afflicted with the dreaded disease.

At least one-half billion per year in lost wages is reported by *The Meridian Star*[2].

Others[3] estimate that 31 million Americans of all ages suffer from arthritis, that it attacks a million new patients a year, and costs the national economy about $15 billion annually[4].

For each male who suffers, there are three females. The symptoms often appear between ages of 20 and 35 with weakness, fever, loss of appetite and weight loss. One or more of the smaller joints becomes inflamed and swollen. Acute, painful inflammation migrates from one joint to another. Mental depression is common.

Attacks may develop gradually, or suddenly with dramatic seizure. Pain and inflammation may come and go for no apparent reason. The disease may affect children and produce stunting of growth and gross deformities.

Considering the insidious nature of rheumatoid diseases, its many forms of symptoms and its long-term degenerative activity on your body, sometimes extending from birth onward, apparently this book is for you, your relatives and your friends!

xi

[1] Davis, K. Carolyne, Letter to Senator James Sasser, September 1, 1982, transmitted by letter to author by Senator James Sasser September 23, 1982.

[2] *The Meridian Star*, "The Arthritis Foundation — Distributing Information to Those with the Affliction" Meridian, MS, February 24, 1983.

[3] *The Scanner*, Volume 1, Number 4, Fall 1981, The Arthritis Institute of the National Hospital for Orthopaedics and Rehabilitation, 2455 Army Navy Drive, Arlington, VA 22206, p. 1.

[4] E. Harrison Clark reports that *Barron's* and *Wall Street Journal* report a figure of $1.5 billion, or a little less for pain-killers.

Chapter I
You and Your So-called Hopeless Disease
For the Rest of Your Life?

So, you've been told you've rheumatic arthritis, and there is no cure! For the rest of your life you must watch your fingers and toes and arms and legs twist and turn and torture themselves into grotesque shapes that offend each eye and spirit!

When you awake each morning your fingers and other joints are swollen, red and they burn as if held to a slow-roasting fire. You flex them and sharp pains make you grimace. Stiffened and puffy, your fingers feel like *not you*, like some burning, sausage-like appendages that were fastened on by instant glue during the night.

Gingerly protecting each joint, you slide carefully from your over-soft mattress. Oh, how it hurts to reach for clothing! Easy now! Not too fast, not too hard! Ouch! How that hurts! You wince, but go on dressing, though slowly. What else can you do?

The Ordinary Made Hard

Someone has tightened the coffee jar lid too much. A flash of resentment stirs as you wonder why others cannot understand, and why they cannot help you more by anticipating your weakness. Again pain forces your immediate attention. It's everywhere, at each joint — the terrible, long-lasting, daily increasing pain. . . .

Dare you risk injury to finger joints by fighting the coffee jar top this morning.

But you *need* the stimulation, the black, warm brew, something — anything — to lighten depression, to sway your outlook. . . .

So you struggle with the cap, gripping down on it, squeezing it and grimacing again, while sharp pains make you want to scream aloud — and then — at last — the jar cap moves ever so slightly. Relaxing your fingers permits pain to diminish somewhat, and then you staunchly tackle the lid again.

You pour the steaming coffee ever so carefully and you hold it even more gingerly. You must not place your fingers about the warm cup, for every finger joint will burn with a fury as though a small, hot laser beam were focussed in them. And so it is with cold items as well. Are you one of those who wisely insulates all cups and glasses?

1

Such are the once easy chores that now loom larger than life itself!

Perhaps you use special tools designed just for invalids with *incurable* arthritis: A wide-band holder for jar caps that multiplies weakened muscles and applies increased friction about the cap; a bathtub grip-bar (what a terrifying experience, that old-fashioned bathtub); an elevated toilet seat; buttoning devices for shirts, coats, blouses; a special device for turning on and off faucets at kitchen or shower (what an absurdly simple act that was once); long handles designed to reach clothing on the floor, and to permit ease in hanging them; special hooks and handles for holding the ever-present coffee cup; a double handle pot holder; special eye and needle affairs for tying shoe-laces — the mechanical devices are endless as the disease works into every muscle-fiber and joint.

Stiffness, Pain, Heat and Cold

How people comment about your hyperactivity! What they don't understand is that if you sit or stand or lay in one position overlong, you become stiff and your joints ache excruciatingly. So you move — here, there, everywhere — all the time!

Do your hands and feet feel cold? Do you sweat night after night, with a terrible burning?

Your walking gait is changing; your skin bruises more easily and it has an increased fragility. Nodules have appeared in skin tissue, especially over points of pressure or friction. If you're bedridden the nodules will be found at the posterior portions of head, trunk and spine.

You might have developed skin ulcers or difficulties of another kind inside your lungs, or any of a dozen other physical problems that at first glance do not appear to be related to arthritis.

But you're probably one of the lucky ones, one of those who can still function, still determine your own physical course daily, still decide for yourself. What of those whose disease has progressed beyond, and now must lie bedridden, or rely on a wheelchair, and must be lifted and towed everywhere, must be dependent upon others, not daily, but hourly, for every little need, every little change, every little pleasure — if any?

Are you still free and financially able to go to a warm climate where blessed relief may temporarily be yours? Oh, how cold rains and winds shrivel us and compress pain upon pain!

2

Hopelessness

Must you lie and stare, and hopelessly dream of the blessings of suicide, the relief of drugs, the wonderful numbness of alcohol . . . , remembering that first visit to your family doctor? "You've rheumatic arthritis and there is no cure. Oh, we know that within the first year you *may* have a spontaneous remission, that perhaps as much as ten to twenty percent of our patients get better. Although sometimes even those have it come and go again.

"Remember, it isn't true that nothing can be done for this disease. Aspirin will kill the pain, and when your system can no longer tolerate aspirin, we've indomethacin, phenylbutazone and many other drugs all designed very nicely to ease inflammation and your pain; we've antimalarial drugs like chloroquine and hydroxychloroquine, and sometimes we use gold compounds, although I wouldn't advise it personally; and there are several others, like propionic acid derivatives and tolmectin . . . .

"Then later, if you do not get better, we may give you cortisone shots — adrenocorticosteroids. I'd not advise that either unless very urgent, as there are dangerous side-effects. . . .

"Don't fret because the majority of patients with rheumatic arthritis can continue to lead active lives with varying degrees of restrictions. We must not seek a short-term solution, but plan for long-range management of your problem.

"There are no specific dietary recommendations[1], but you should maintain a good balanced diet, and there are no indications of vitamin supplementation, unless, of course, you just happen to have a special vitamin problem, which I don't believe is true for you. Weight reduction — and keeping it off — should have a high priority.

"You must have rest, and we must determine a program of maintenance of joint function by physical measures, and also we don't want your muscles to atrophy. In other words some kinds of exercises are a must, so long as you don't over-stress your joints.

"Then there is the inevitable depression and fatigue. . . . "

"Depression?" you ask. "Fatigue?"

Do you need a lecture on depression and fatigue?

Sharp and dull pains bombard your each waking moment, until there is nothing left but for your analytical mind to attenuate, to close down, to push you into a state of emotional apathy that is beyond words.

3

Nothing, absolutely nothing on earth or beyond earth, can have meaning when you are at lowest ebb. Loved ones speak, and you groan, or turn-over, or at the very best you growl out, "I just don't give a damn!" and you mean it with every cell, every fiber of your being. Your spouse could move out at that instance, and you'd care not! Your beautiful children could be crying of ache and loneliness, and you'd care not! Your house might be leaking, or in danger of burning down, and you'd care not! You could be told of inheriting a million dollars, and you'd care not! A flying saucer could land beside your bedroom window emitting five little green men, each carrying strange weapons that will evaporate anything they touch, and you'd care not!

You could die at that instant, and you'd care not!

Please physician, tell us about apathy and fatigue. . . .

Traditional Treatments

But the body recovers with rest, although with lessened vigor at each interval, and morning comes again. You struggle to dress, to remove the coffee jar lid, to move about, and to bathe and go through the motions of easing your daily load.

Time passes. Another trip to the doctor, and another. Your medicine closet bulges: besides aspirin there is now Indocin®, Butazolidin®, Motrin®, Clinoril®, Tolectin®, Naprosyn®, Feldene®. Each day you take one or another with increased frequency.

You may be one of those whose system rebels further, and you may suffer eternal diarrhea, or you may have developed stomach ulcers, or some other insidious problem — just when you thought your body withstood all the problems it could bear. . . !

Little by little, over weeks and months, you watch fingers and toes turn and bend, despite rigorous exercises, and you constantly fight pain. There is absolutely nothing that can be done, except now and then expensive physical therapy might slow the terrible deformation if conducted under proper professional conditions, — but eventually nothing helps when the very joints and cartilages and tendons themselves have been eaten alive.

Now you've become a ranking candidate for prosthesis, those wonderful steel and plastic devices that are transplanted into joints.

Terrible you say?

Not so! Not if your life consists of unmoving, continuous

staring at a colorless, lifeless ceiling above your bed, and a terrible moment by moment waiting for someone to come and move you from hither to thither.

Joint by joint is destroyed by the raging inferno of your own immunological system, your life eating up yourself, and joint by joint can, perhaps, be replaced, until there is little *you* left at all, or until you finally, blessedly, succumb to the greatest depression of all — death!

You are probably intelligent enough to know your future — *you've seen so many others with this terrifying sickness.* You've got choices. You can fight, do all the things your family doctor tells you to do: keep down inflammation and pain; exercise, but also rest frequently.

Non-traditional Treatments

Or, like so many of us, you can ignore medical science and technical knowledge and react to hearsay, superstition, panaceas. You know! Copper bracelets[2]; cactus juice[3]; special diets; faith healers; mumbo-jumbo of one kind or another.

Who can blame us?

There is no hope, because there is no known cause, we've been told; and every day the depression and pain and fatigue and weakness increases, as does the bending and twisting and distortion of ourselves.

You look in the faces of loved ones, spouses and children and grandchildren, who move with gay abandon and carrry on life with zest that was once yours — and you wonder — can you impose this frightful crippling burden on their wonderful future? Do you have the right? Do they have the obligation to suffer with you?

What kind of terrible sin have you committed, you secretly wonder, *that the Lord put this on. . . ?*

Somewhere secretly deep inside you've committed yourself to ending it all at just the right time if you can find a way to do so *without hurting them.*

Meanwhile, any hope, *something* is better than *nothing at all,* even if that something is simply *fantasized hope!* Who would take that away also?

So there is nothing you can do!

Live with it, and search for relief anywhere, everywhere, and hope or give up life completely — that's our choice!

5

So we search in national newspapers for special arthritis cures — if you don't like this week's, there's always another coming along next week just to keep our fantasies alive; we look into fancy diet books and magazines and organic health journals; we carefully listen to positive sounding, authoritarian faith healers, those men who are so sure that if we will just *believe* a higher power will reach out with a mystical touch and lo! we are healed; oh, how we donate to their favorite causes; and we drink this briny juice, or eat that tasteless herb, or we go on special diets that would normally make us very happy if we were herbivores; or we spend time and much money getting ourselves analyzed and explained away by one school of head-shrinks or another. . . .

No matter, all the time the terrible fires rage, our joints puff and shriek with pain, and the inexorable horrible twisting and turning marches onward!

So Where From Here?

So here you are now, with this publication, with just another claim to cure. You're pessimistic, aren't you? *You have a right to be.* So, keep your pessimism.

If what follows makes sense, you'll try it, like you've tried so many other things that didn't work, even when they didn't make sense. If it is science, if it is proper medical practice, it'll work. If it works, you'll be well. If it doesn't work, you're no worse off, especially since the time and cost involved in this alleged "real cure" is relatively tiny, and especially since your own family doctor can be party to the cure.

What have you to lose? A six weeks trial at very little cost under your own family physician?

That's not much compared to an endless lifetime draining cacti of their sap, or eating alfalfa, or doing some other silly thing, is it?

Read on, if you dare, if you can stand one more hope.

And God be good to you as he has already been good to so many others. . . .

---

[1] Advice from some physicians differ. Dr. Robert Bingham, for example, states that 60% of rheumatoid arthritis patients have dietary deficiencies, and 80% have vitamin and mineral deficiencies.

[2] According to Professor Roger Wyburn-Mason, copper ions from a copper bracelet, on invading the bloodstream, can in fact weaken an amoebic infection which is the primary source cause of rheumatoid arthritis; but that the copper ion concentration

from a bracelet source is not usually sufficient to reduce the infective population in the drastic numbers necessary.

[3] According to Dr. Robert Bingham, Yucca juice is helpful for *some* rheumatoid arthritis patients. Its usefulness seems to come from its two most important chemical components: saponin, which facilitates the combination of oil and water aiding digestion and elimination, the other a vegetable steroid related to the cortisone family of drugs, thereby relieving symptoms.

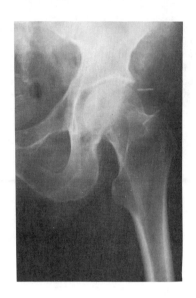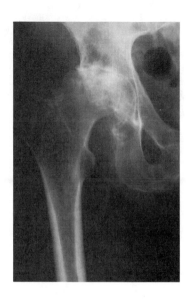

(On left) Left hip joint of Jack M. Blount, M.D., which shows normal head and acetabulum (socket). (On Right) Right hip joint of Jack M. Blount, M.D., which shows abnormal (fragmented) head and acetabulum (socket) caused by rheumatoid disease (aseptic necrosis). X-rays taken December 11, 1975.

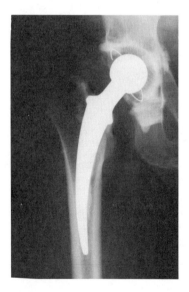

Right hip joint of Jack M. Blount, M.D., showing Charnley's prosthetic implant and acrylic socket, March 21, 1976.

Chapter II
Dr. Jack M. Blount's "Miracle"
Dr. Jack M. Blount's Gift to Mankind

Dr. Jack M. Blount's story is an emotionally gripping account of a man who has been to the very depths of hell and has come back to tell us how he escaped the fires. He tells his story simply, without any attempt to embellish, and it is told with a genuineness that makes you believe in his continued concern for your health and welfare. In this chapter Dr. Blount will tell his own story in his own words. Keep in mind that he is cured of the ravages of rheumatoid arthritis, that he has since treated better than 16,000 patients successfully, and that he freely gives of his knowledge to any who ask. He is a man who was active physically in his youth although his symptoms began as a systemic illness in his teens with muscle pain, metatarsalgia (pain in the foot), lumbago (pain in the back), intercostal (between ribs) pains, iridocyclitis (inflammation of eye), psoriasis (skin lesions) and that eventually he got pains in the joints, generalized arthritis with effusions (fluids into joints), carpal tunnel syndrome (compression of nerve in wrist), paresthesia (loss of feeling or perverted sensation), ulcerative colitis (sore or inflammation of colon), aseptic necrosis (death) of a femoral head for which a prothesis (steel and plastic joint) was inserted, etc. He was reduced to total invalidism and took to alcohol, morphine-containing drugs, barbiturates and was a terminal case. He had to give up his medical practice in March 1974 and had taken steroids for more than twenty years.

Dr. Blount's Story: Rheumatoid Disease
is of the Entire Body

I cured myself and more than 16,000 others of an incurable illness. RHEUMATOID DISEASE. I call it a MIRACLE.

I had rheumatoid disease. Rheumatoid disease is a disease of the entire body, not of just the joints, although most of the pain and destruction seems to be in and around the joints. I was hopelessly ill.

In the Spring of 1974 I had developed aseptic necrosis (complete destruction) of my right hip socket and femoral head. I had to quit work (private medical practice) and take to the bed. The only thing that would help was a hip replacement with a prosthesis. The orthopedic surgeon that I went to said at first he would do the operation but then changed his mind giving the excuse that because I was only fifty-two years old at the time I was ineligible. They didn't know, yet, how much dependence to put on procedure.

Despair

Despair set in, I could only lie in bed and stare at the ceiling. The cure of my illness was hopeless. No one knew the cause. No one knew anything useful to do for it. The usual advice was to take a lot of aspirin and learn to live with it. Pharmaceutical companies tried to improve on aspirin and gave us Butazolidin®, Indocin®, Motrin®, Tolectin®, Nalfon®, Naprosyn®, Clinoril®, Meclomen®, etc. They called these *"nonsteroidal anti-inflammatory"* agents: all were useless except for some analgesic effect.

"Cortisone" was introduced in 1949 and was hailed for a while as the long awaited answer. It was, and still is, the quickest relief of arthritis symptoms, but it causes devastation worse than the disease. These adverse effects included hyperadrenalism (Cushing's Disease) diabetes, ulcers, weakened bone, (decalcification) etc. I took a form of this for about twenty years.

While lying in bed my arthritis became complicated by colitis, with diarrhea of sometimes up to twenty times a day, kidney stones, alcohol, and drugs. I was in and out of hospitals repeatedly. I thought I would surely die. Friends kept sending word that they were praying for me. I often thought of committing suicide. The pain and agony were unbearable. One morning after I had accumulated about forty Seconal® capsules (sleeping pills) I swallowed them all. Four have been known to kill. I didn't want to kill myself, but I couldn't endure such perpetual agony. After some hours my wife found me unconscious and on finding the empty bottle, she knew what I had done. I awoke very groggy and tied to a hospital bed. After regaining enough sense to know anything at all, I wanted to know if I had been apneic. (Had I been deprived of oxygen long enough to cause permanent brain damage?) I was assured the answer was "no." Despite such an overwhelming dose of sleeping pills I had continued to breathe adequately without supplemental oxygen or assisted breathing. This was a miracle in itself. "Somebody up There" was not ready for me.

Why Was I Saved?

Back home I kept breathing but hardly living. Why was I still

10

here at all? I had been waiting for some earthly savior and none came. Was there some "learned University professor or researcher" somewhere who knew something to do?

The Miracle of Professor Roger Wyburn-Mason

One day in the spring of 1976 I came across an article in *Modern Medicine*[1] entitled "Rheumatoid Disease: Has One Man Found the Cause and Cure of Rheumatoid Disease? Arthritis," written by Robert Bingham, M.D., practicing in Riverside County, California. Dr. Bingham, orthopedic surgeon, had heard of work done by Professor Roger Wyburn-Mason, Richmond Hill, Surrey, England, and had gone to England to interview the Professor. His article told about how the English researcher, practitioner, microbiologist, had determined that the etiological agent (cause) of rheumatoid disease is actually a germ, a protozoon, an amoeba, similar to the "lettuce bug" amoeba that causes dysentery. He also reported that a chemical (in fact, several chemicals) had been found that would kill the "bug" in patients without killing the patient.

He was curing people who had the disease that was killing me. The chemical (medicine) that the Professor was using successfully was called *clotrimazole*.

That's wonderful, but how could I get some for myself? It was not and still is not on the market anywhere in the world for systemic use.

Finally, in the Spring of 1976, my orthopedic surgeon decided to operate. They removed the upper part of the right femur with the femoral head and reamed out the acetabulum (socket). The socket was filled in with plastic to make a new one and the bone was replaced with a "comma-shaped" steel rod with the pointed end inserted down into the marrow, distally, of the remaining femur.

Now, I thought I would recover. But recovery was terrible. I still needed my pain medicine and booze. My brother became disgusted with me and had me sent to an alcoholic ward and "detox" center at the State Hospital. After a month there I was off everything addicting except my daily early morning "Cortisone." I still had my rheumatoid disease — my germs, the amoeba. I still had to rid my body of them. The operation seemed to give them new life.

11

Somehow, I remembered that *clotrimazole* is the active ingredient in a preparation used to treat yeast and fungus infections of the skin but it was just one part *clotrimazole* plus ninety-nine parts propelene glycol, car antifreeze — Prestone®. This is poisonous to man if taken internally. I decided to telephone Delbay, the company that puts the mixture together, and see if I could get *clotrimazole* that hadn't been mixed. The answer was "no." They were afraid of the U.S. Food and Drug Administration.

Failing with that endeavor I started wondering if there might be something else almost the same that would work. I looked at the word *clotrimazole* and focused on the *azole*. I looked that up in the medical dictionary and found that the parent of this is *Imidazole*. Somehow I remembered that I had heard that word somewhere before. I kept repeating it. Then I remembered that this is the chemical name of the medicine *metronidazole*, or *Flagyl®*. I compared the formulas of the two and they looked close enough alike that I thought it was worth a trial. We had had *Flagyl®* since 1962 and used it to cure amebiasis (intestinal) and vaginal trichomonas infections. It was known to be able to kill both of these protozoa. I decided to try it. Later I pulled out a drawer in my bath room and there was a bottle of one hundred *Flagyl®* tablets. A MIRACLE! God had put the answer to my illness that close to me.

How should I take it? I realized that the small dosages that were recommended for trichomonas and intestinal amebiasis would not do any good. If it would have, someone would have discovered it accidentally. I checked the medical text books and saw that it had been given in doses as high as three tablets, 250 mgm, three times daily. That is the amount I started to take.

I Experiment On Myself

I didn't know how long to continue taking it. I didn't know if it would kill me. I realized I didn't have much to lose; therefore I took all I had which lasted eleven days. On the morning of the eleventh day, I got nauseated while brushing my teeth — and emptied my stomach. Then I knew I couldn't take anymore even if I had had more readily available, so I stopped.

But during these eleven days a miracle had begun to happen. My arthritis started getting better. I awoke in the middle of the night and realized that the soreness, stiffness, and swelling had started subsiding. I looked at my hands which had been so bad and now were so much better. I couldn't hold back the tears. I started praying and thanking God.

After that I didn't know how much was enough. I knew that I was still sick. I still had sweats and felt cold. I was bound to still have the infection. After two weeks I decided that I needed more. I restarted taking three 250 mgm tablets three times a day. I took it for eleven days more and on the eleventh day I got nauseated again. But, I was surely improving by the day. I decided to continue this pattern.

More Successful Patients

I decided to find out if some of my former arthritis patients were brave enough to try it.

I telephoned them and invited several of them to my home, one at a time. To each I explained what it was all about. Every single one was eager to try it, nothing else had ever helped. Why not? During the Summer of 1977 about thirty of them were treated and most of them had the same good experience that I had. Some got nauseated from the start and decided to quit.

Among the thirty was a Reverend Ethel Beall. Brother Beall not only had arthritis, but had lost a leg due to an automobile accident. The bone in the stump of the leg had gotten infected and drained constantly and was always painful. During this treatment period with *Flagyl*® his arthritis got better and his leg got well and stopped hurting. (Several months later he died suddenly of embolus [blood clot] while recovering from a prostate operation).

Well Again!

After 8 months I was able to return to my private medical practice on a limited basis. I had been out three and one-half years. On September 1st 1977, I was back in the office seeing patients by appointments.

I decided to write Professor Roger Wyburn-Mason in England and tell him of my experiences. I owed him my life. He answered immediately and said that he had decided to include my case in a book he was writing. *The Causation of Rheumatoid Disease and Many Human Cancers — A New Concept in Medicine.* My story appears on page 205 in the book, which was published in Japan in March 1978 by a Professor T. Koba, who obtained the original manuscript from Professor Wyburn-Mason[2].

We continue to correspond and I visited with him during the

13

Summer of 1978. He told me that he tried metronidazole at one time and it didn't work. His dosage was not adequate; he had tried giving only 250 mgm three times daily. However, later he gave 750 mgm three times daily and it did work about equally as well as *clotrimazole*. He found other *nitroimidazoles* that would do the job, also.

Lately he has found three commonly used medications that are amoebicidal when used in high doses: furazolidone, allopurinol and rifampicin.

His experiments proved that *Flagyl*® and the other *nitroimidazoles* are excreted slowly from the body and it is not necessary to give them on a daily basis. After giving a loading dose for two days there is an effective blood level (for killing the amoebae) for several days more. During the past six years I have treated more than 16,000 arthritic people with very gratifying results. Some are cured of the disease while in others it has been arrested. People are now coming from all over to share in this miracle.

Professor Roger Wyburn-Mason should be nominated for the *Nobel Prize* in medicine.

Prayer for the Entire World

I pray that the entire world will soon know and people every where can receive the same relief that I have. What a joy I know now!

I thank God!

This information is free to whomever will take and use it. I *need* no wealth and *seek* no fame.

---

[1] *Modern Medicine*, "Rheumatoid Disease: Has One Investigator Found Its Cause and Its Cure?" Robert Bingham, M.D., Feb. 15, 1976, pp. 38-47.

[2] Published by Iji Publishing Co., Ltd., Japan ($125). Out of print. Limited number have been donated to medical libraries (USA) by Jack M. Blount, Jr., M.D. *Addenda* (precis' and summary) available from *The Rheumatoid Disease Foundation* ($7.50 plus $1.00 postage and handling); also write for information on loan copies of basic work.

Important Note

William Renforth, M.D. (Connersville, IN, USA) deserves respectful praise for research of nitroimidazoles prior to 1977, distributing information and pioneering in the use of metronidazole for treatment of Rheumatoid Disease. Dr. Archimedes Concon (Memphis, TN) following a non-amoebic theory, also effectively used metronidazole for RD prior to 1976. [From time to time historically important papers will be published by *The Rheumatoid Disease Foundation*.]

Chapter III
The Author is Also Cured

The Beginning of Arthritis

In 1978 the author, at age 53, began suffering from the first pangs of rheumatoid arthritis, although at the time it was passed off as simply unimportant, transitory pains in toes and fingers and groin of unknown origin.

By choice the author slept on a hard, cotton-pad, but slowly shoulder pains became so great that foam padding had to be overlayed.

Later visits to medical specialists brought out that the pains were from "degenerative arthritis." This diagnosis was confirmed by medical doctors at the Veteran's Administration Hospital.

Fatigue and Depression

During the following year the author began experiencing a kind of fatigue that sapped strength and made for a hopeless despair at times which was never part of his former life. Considering the fact that the author had normally worked more than one job or position, had stayed busy seven days a week writing or teaching, or working about the yard and house, and now he was listless and suffering periodic bouts of almost complete apathy, it became clear early that something more serious was wrong. During one of these severe periods, when apathy was deepest, a misunderstanding with spouse triggered off a divorce after thirty years of marriage and ten children.

Since there seemed to be a medically defined distinction between rheumatoid arthritis and degenerative arthritis, and the writer was told (wrongly) that the former required considerable more rest and the second required active exercise of a moderate nature, this writer undertook to begin learning to play the piano and to also dance.

There's little question that the various physical exercises kept joints fluid[1], although painfully so at times, but the greatest puzzle was in the fact that within two years of the initial diagnosis of "degenerative" arthritis, the small finger on the right hand began to turn sidewise, and a typical rheumatoid arthritis and hard nodule had begun to form at this joint.

Pains Increase

Pains continued to increase at various joints, and finally, about three years into the disease, the hands began to flush red and hot and to swell, especially on arising early mornings. A great number of like symptoms lasted throughout the day.

It became almost impossible to type on the author's regular manual typewriter, because of pain kick-back to the joints.

Now the little finger on the left hand began to twist also, and all the joints at the hands began to almost glow a firey red.

The author was having difficulty opening ordinary bottles: catchup, pickle jars, soft drink; and the problem of opening sacks of peanuts became a procedure of first cutting the celluloid wrappings with a knife, instead of gripping and tearing with fingers.

Lifting pots and pans became an exceedingly painful chore.

Changing a tire without help was excruciatingly difficult.

His children could not understand why the author's habits had changed so drastically. Once there was nothing he would ask them to do in the way of farm or house maintenance that he, himself, would not chip in to do.

Hopelessness extended from self to family to friends, and finally even to passing acquaintances who could instinctively sense the unhappiness carried about by this rapidly aging man.

How could one make fast friends when daily his body was changing, and daily one became weaker and more ineffective with everything touched?

How could long-range committments be kept, or strong personal relations be acknowledged? How fair is it to impose on those you love such burdens: future helplessness and twisted grotesqueness?

The author was sufficiently imaginative to know where it would end, and frankly did not want to burden anyone with what was coming. He would rather be dead than crippled and helpless and apathetic and sapping the youth and vitality of his children.

Still, the author, having had an extensive scientific background (mathematics, chemistry, physics, psychology) and also a very wide-ranging background in many different disciplines, started searching through technical literature (just as did Dr. Blount) and talking to people. Only by fortuitous accident did he come to be helped by Dr. Jack M. Blount, and it came about through this series of connections:

The Discovery

A daughter-in-law knew of the author's terrible pains and his search in the literature. She mentioned the author's search to parents. They had a friend who'd been to Dr. Blount and had been cured. They suggested to her that her father-in-law write to Dr. Blount.

Like so many others in like predicament, the author sent out the letter, not with great anticipation — frankly he thought he'd be fluffed off to his family doctor — but because by now (as those with the condition know) one cannot afford to overlook anything.

Lo! A most amazing answer came back, consisting of three pages, that described Dr. Blount's own search and cure, as told in Chapter II above, and in that correspondence was embedded the name and amount of the drug necessary to produce the cure — *at no expense to the author.*

The Cure

The author tried Dr. Blount's treatment, which lasted six weeks. Here's what happened:

- After two weeks the puffiness and redness of fingers disappeared for the first time in a half year.
- After four weeks the pain, depression and fatigue ended.
- After seven weeks the redness of finger joints nearly disappeared.
- After seven weeks the author's attitude toward life and people changed remarkably, and again he feels like life is worth the effort, and so are people and personal relations.

There are still problems. The twisted little fingers are still distorted, and they still hurt when used. Damaged joints may never heal, but where capillaries exist, over time, healing may again proceed faster than self-destruction. There is some redness of the other finger joints from time to time, especially when used for long periods at the typewriter. There is still some pain of other joints here and there. Dr. Blount says that experience shows most of these residual pains will settle out in time.

But, the author can daily turn more bottle tops, and lift heavier loads, and wrestle playfully with another without screaming bloody murder!

And best of all extreme apathy is gone, as is middle-of-day fatigue!

Can there be a better gift from one human to another, than this, that health and happiness is restored, and at no cost, except that of minor medicines?

Need the author state: *I love Dr. Jack Blount and Professor Roger Wyburn-Mason, the first for courage, fortitude and charity, the second for wisdom, persistence and intelligence!*

---

[1] According to Professor Roger Wyburn-Mason, all forms of arthritis should be rested, as joint activity increases inflammation and pain and prevents healing.

Chapter IV
The "MIRACLE" Treatment

Recommended Treatments
To your family doctor, we say:
Antiamoebics have never been considered for use against rheumatoid diseases because the various arthritis associations have not yet investigated Professor Roger Wyburn-Mason's brilliant scientific work, published now since 1964.
You must decide if the prescriptions that follow are harmful to your patient. If not, is the cost involved worth a trial, considering the hopeless and insidious nature of the diseases?
Many cooperating physicians are using the protocol that follows:

The Roger Wyburn-Mason
&
Jack M. Blount Foundation
for Eradication of Rheumatoid Disease
Rt. 4, Box 137 § Franklin, TN 37064 § *(615) 646-1030*
"The Rheumatoid Disease Foundation"
A non-profit, charitable, tax-exempt organization

The Rheumatoid Disease Foundation, through its cooperating physicians in a committee chaired by Robert Johnson, M.D. (Charleston, SC) has established the following standards of practice when treating rheumatoid disease. These are suggested standards. Many physicians will exceed these basic standards. What follows is an outline developed through research and experience of cooperating physicians. A SIMPLE AND INEXPENSIVE CURE/REMISSION FOR RHEUMATOID DISEASES IS SET OUT IN WHAT FOLLOWS. DRAW YOUR DOCTOR'S ATTENTION TO THE MEDICATIONS THAT OTHER PHYSICIANS ARE ALREADY USING EFFECTIVELY. IF YOU DO NOT HAVE A FAMILY DOCTOR, WRITE FOR OUR LIST OF COOPERATING PHYSICIANS.

Your family physician should know that there are at least two genus of limax amoeba (one-celled animal life) that cause Rheumatoid Disease if you are genetically susceptible to it, or its products: Acanthamoeba and/or Naegleria.

Within these two genus are many species, and strains within species, and they vary considerably in their ability to adapt to various antiprotozoal agents. Where one antiamoebic will kill one organism inside the body, another will not, and which organism affects you can only be learned by trial and error. Success rates from the first application of the treatment program listed below varies from 78% to 95% depending on which physician and which group of patients is being treated. The success rate is higher whenever further applications of the appropriate antiamoebic is used.

If the first treatment does not bring about a Herxheimer reaction, the physician is advised to move to another antiamoebic, and in any case, both this *Foundation* as well as any of the cooperating physicians will be more than happy to share their experiences.

The Foundation cannot, of course, be responsible for mal-application, mis-application, or inappropriate treatment of any kind, and again suggests that all treatment, if possible, be through your family physician.

19

Rheumatoid Disease Protocol

The central theme of treatment is based on the preliminary work of Professor Roger Wyburn-Mason and Jack M. Blount, M.D. and later findings of Robert Bingham, M.D.; it also seeks to introduce physicians to alternative or extended courses of treatment that have been found to be useful by other physicians in the organization, the goals being to: (1) arrest rheumatoid disease, (2) repair damage caused by rheumatoid disease, (3) further the maintenance of wellness.

This protocol is intended as an outline, and cannot serve as a "course in treatment" for rheumatoid disease. It is necessary for each physician to pursue his/her own intricacies of modalities mentioned.

I. Diagnosis: shall be made on the basis of
- **A. Patient History — to include**
   1. Time of onset
   2. Degree of disability
   3. Family history
   4. Remissions and exacerbations
   5. Contributing factors
   6. Previous treatment modalities and results thereof
   7. Activity pattern
   8. Medications being taken
- **B. Physical Examination**
   1. General appearance
   2. Weight and height
   3. Blood pressure and pulse
   4. Head and neck
   5. Cardio-vascular system
   6. Abdomen
   7. Musculo-skeletal system (to include evaluation of joints)
- **C. Laboratory testing**
   1. Urinalysis
   2. SMAC-24
   3. Rheumatoid panel (to include sedimentation rate and CRP)
   4. Analysis of synovial fluid (when present)
   5. Other (as indicated)
   6. Electrocardiogram
   7. X-rays of affected joints (if indicated)
   8. Any of the above that have been performed by another physician within the past 60 days may be utilized at the discretion of the treating physician.

II. Treatment: (several treatment regimens are available)
- **A. Oral medications**
   1. Nitroimidazoles
      (a). Metronidazole
      (b). Tinidazole
      (c). Clotrimazole
      Whichever nitroimidazole is used, the dosage (modified by weight) is the same: 2 grams daily for two (2) days each week X6 weeks. (**Children: 250mg/25 pounds body weight**).
   2. Furazolidone (Furoxone) 100 mgm q.i.d. X1 week
   3. Iodoquinol 650 mgm t.i.d. X3 weeks
   4. POTABA 2 grams 6 times daily X2 weeks
   5. Allopurinol 300 mgm t.i.d. X1 week (**this in conjunction with one of the**

20

above 5 antiamoebics — 1.(a), 1. (b), 1.(c),2, 3. — used together acts as broad spectrum antiamoebic).
  6. Rifampin or Rimactane 600 mgm daily X1 month **(If reactions are severe, stop treatment immediately)**.
B. Injections
  1. Intraneural Injections (technique of Dr. Paul K. Pybus, Dr. I.H.J. Bourne)
  2. Cleveland Clinic treatment (method of Jack M. Blount, M.D.: Lumbar subarachnoid injection of 2.5 cc of 0.3% procaine with 20 mgm Depo-Medrol)
C. Nutrition (to include vitamin and mineral supplements as well as counseling relative to diet).
D. Steroids — the use of prednisone 20 mgm daily X5 days or Depo-Medrol 40 mgm injection X1 will reduce considerably the Jarisch-Herxheimer reaction often seen when initiating therapy (See General Information).
E. Ancillary treatment modalities (as used by various advisory committee members).
  1. Mega vitamin dosage (Prosch, Reich, Bingham)
  2. Chelation therapy (American Academy of Medical Preventics — AAMPS)
  3. Hot mineral baths (Bingham)
F. Return visits
  1. Return visits should probably be in 1 week, 3 weeks, 6 weeks, then every 3 months thereafter.
  2. Preventive maintenance: It usually helps to prevent the recurrence of rheumatoid disease if the patient is given a round of treatment with allopurinol at 6 months post original treatment and every 6 months thereafter. If symptoms are present, the entire original treatment regimen should be repeated. **(Allopurinol can cause a very severe reaction on the second round of treatment** — Wyburn-Mason).
G. General Information
  1. Most patients will need counseling about diet and nutrition.
  2. Explanation of the Jarisch-Herxheimer reaction often will prevent patient drop-out in many cases.
  3. Since Metronidazole is the only nitroimidazole currently available in the United States, it is probably the drug of choice for beginning treatment.
  4. Utilization of the "Cleveland Clinic" injection and intraneural injections should probably be reserved until the individual physician has had the opportunity to learn the technique from a physician already using it.
  5. Most of the foregoing treatment is directed toward rheumatoid disease. Osteoarthritis has been found to respond much less dramatically, although it does often show some degree of improvement. (Best results seem to be achieved with intraneural injections.)
  6. Rationale for treatment with antiamoebics: Based on Dr. Roger Wyburn-Mason's work which demonstrated free-living limax amoeba to be the causative agent in rheumatoid disease, amoebicidal drugs have been postulated as a treatment of choice. When these drugs kill the organism, the release of foreign proteins usually results in a Jarisch-Herxheimer reaction (similar to the old arsenical treatment for syphilis). This results in a temporary generalized increase of rheumatoid symptoms with the administration of an antirheumatic drug.
  7. Drug reactions
    (a). Rifampicin — violent Herxheimer. In this event, discontinue treatment with rifampicin at once.
    (b). Allopurinol — leg pain, temperature spike, chills, sweating, rash on body and face.

This protocol is subject to revisions (additions, deletions, changes) as *The Rheumatoid Disease Foundation* completes relevant research.

Perry A. Chapdelaine, Sr.
Executive Director/Secretary
Revised 1985: Physicians & Scientists Committee

Since alcohol in presence of antiamoebics (*metronidazole, allopurinol*) (or antibiotics) makes some people sick, it may be best not to take any alcohol during period of treatment of six weeks. (The medicine will stay in the body during the first four weeks.) Also sometimes alcohol destroys certain chemical compounds; and, in the case of several antiamoebics, alcohol is definitely not a good idea.

If you are taking other medicines, such as anti-inflammatory drugs for arthritis, and other than cortisone compounds, you may continue taking them. There will be no conflicting side-effects. However, for the most part, it is best if you *check with your family physician when determining possible contra-indications of other medicines.*

Cost of these medicines may vary from $37 to several hundred dollars depending upon your treatment, the pharmacy with which you trade, and the length of time you are treated.

Please keep in mind that every physician including your own will have additional treatment modalities in mind: nutritional guidance, exercise, strengthening of the immunological system by various techniques, chelation therapy, hot baths, and so on. You should understand what your treatment will consist of in advance, and why, before rejecting your physician's directions out of hand.

However, in no case should you permit the use of gold shot's or penicillamine at the same time you are taking antiamoebics.

The response of patients to the above medicines is often inhibited by long-continued, previous treatment with gold injections, penicillamine or corticosteroids[3]. Each patient must be considered and studied independently, for the most effective treatment.

And while the former use of gold shots and/or penicillamine does not necessarily mean that you will not respond (many do), it may mean that you must find a way to chelate out the residual gold prior to having effective antiamoebic treatment.

F.M. Logsdon, M.D. (TX: deceased) developed a technique that seemed effective using the American Academy of Medical Preventics (AAMPS) treatment protocol for chelating out residual gold, following the progress through several chelations via laboratory tests.

On the Herxheimer

From experience, your primary rheumatoid arthritic symptoms should begin to be alleviated within a day or so, although it is not unusual for several weeks to go by before changes are observed.

In particular, *one should know that the fever and swollen feeling and appearance of joints may be increased at first*. The symptoms may appear very similar to flu symptoms: flushing of skin, sweating, aching bones, fever, headache, sometimes running nose . . . like a foreign protein reaction. This is the Jarisch-Herxheimer reaction which is a "transiently increased discomfort in skin lesions and temperature elevations occurring . . . after start of antiamoebic treatment . . . " according to a medical dictionary.

You may also be quite allergic to the proteins (and/or the toxic products) of the rapidly dying protozoa that swarm in your body and the Jarisch-Herxheimer reaction is related to that "allergy," a phenomenon very similar to a serum reaction.

However, despair not! Within days to weeks at most, this reaction (if you have it) will be lessened, and you will be pleasantly surprised!

The use of antiamoebics for treatment of Rheumatoid Diseases was introduced by Roger Wyburn-Mason in 1964 in the Henry Kimpton/Charles C. Thomas publication, *A New Protozoon* and also at the IXth International Conference of Chemotherapy held in London, England in July 1975.

Chief antiamoebics recommended by *The Rheumatoid Disease Foundation* are imidazoles where substitution has been made in the ONE position (Dr. John R.A. Simoons, Pharmacology).

These compounds are amoebicidal *in vitro* against species of *Naegleria* and *Acanthamoeba*.

Metronidazole does not fit in the above classification, and is not amoebicidal *in vitro* against the named genus. Since Metronidazole works *in vivo* we speculate that one of its two chief metabolites, both azoles, and resulting from intestinal bacterial action, may be the active substance(s). (Metronidazole is the only nitroimidazole available in the United States). Antibiotics, of course, can knock out desirable microflora.

Wojtulewski evaluated clotrimazole in a double-blind study, finding this compound "effective in the treatment of Rheumatoid Arthritis and superior to Ketoprofen." ("Clotrimazole in Rheumatoid Arthritis," *Annals of the Rheumatic Diseases*, 1980, 39, 469-472.)

The Rheumatoid Disease Foundation is funding placebo controlled, double-blind studies at Bowman Gray School of Medicine, Wake Forest University, Winston-Salem, NC (Chief Investigator, Robert A. Turner, M.D., Chief, Rheumatology Section).

The Rheumatoid Disease Foundation, following the life-time work of Professor Roger Wyburn-Mason, views Rheumatoid Disease as consisting of perhaps more than 100 different presenting symptoms, depending upon which tissues are affected by which genus, species, or strain of limax amoeba. Key to understanding the treatment protocol is observing the Jarisch-Herxheimer effect (flu-like-symptoms) accompanying the use of antiamoebics. When treating Leprosy, the phenomenon is known as Lucio's Phenomenon. Treatment of tuberculosis, and the historical arsenical treatment of syphilis creates the same phenomenon.

While *The Rheumatoid Disease Foundation* views the limax amoeba theory as being the most probable (and workable) hypothesis in explaining and bringing about cure/remission of Rheumatoid Diseases, it recognizes that a multiplicity of factors are at work, including genetic susceptibility, nutrition and other good health rules; and it does not view free-radical explanations as being inconsistent with the limax amoeba hypothesis.

One difficulty seen in hindsight has been in distinguishing between the disease as an on-going process and the damage done by the disease.

The disease can be stopped but many of the symptoms having resulted from the disease — the damage done — may prevail, requiring other treatment protocols: nutrition, chelation, exercise, surgery, et. al.

Open studies, using various antiamoebics in the treatment of Rheumatoid Diseases by Drs. Robert Bingham, Gus J. Prosch, Jr., Paul K. Pybus depict results varying from 78% to 95%. [Anna Boland's, M.D. (Korea) figures are less while Seldon Nelson's, D.O. (Michigan) are more]

Traditional, anticipated placebo effects in an open study would not be greater than about 33%. Results showing 78-95% are considerably beyond placebo expectations.

[Wyburn-Mason/Pybus intraneural injection studies show excellent results when treating pains of Rheumatoid Disease and Osteoarthritis. Additional independently conceived and developed intraneural injection studies are available from Dr. I.H.J. Bourne (Richmond, Thorndon Approach, Herongate, Brentwood CM 13 3PA, England).]

In a letter to Dr. John R.A. Simoons, July 7, 1984, Gus J. Prosch, Jr., M.D. says:

Let me make some general statements concerning past observations and studies that I have concluded to be the truth in treating Rheumatoid Disease with antiamoebic drugs.

1. I recently completed a research project concerning the treating of 200 patients with Rheumatoid Disease with antiamoebic medication. The primary antiamoebic used was Metronidazole and when the desired response was not forthcoming I used other antiamoebics such as Allopurinol, Furazolidone or Rimactane. Final analysis demonstrated 78% good to excellent (cured or in remission) results and 22% showing

poor to no result. All patients having a favorable response had some Herxheimer reaction and those showing poor to no response demonstrated very mild to no Herxheimer reaction. Incidentally, no serious side effects were observed from the medication.

2. The amoeba (or offending agent) can involve (or infect) *any* body tissue, organ or system.

3. If involved (or infected) that tissue, organ or system can demonstrate some form of a Herxheimer reaction when antiamoebic medication is introduced into the body.

4. With the initial introduction (1st week) of the antiamoebic medication, the Herxheimer reaction can be so severe that patients become fearful that the medication is doing them great harm and may want to stop the treatment. For this reason a single initial injection of 20-40 mg of Depot Medrol is usually given to lessen the severity of the reaction.

5. After the second week of medication, the reaction gradually begins to subside, as fewer amoebae (or offending germ or agent) are killed and less antigen is released in the body.

6. If a patient has *any* Herxheimer reaction following the sixth week of medication, the patient is still infected and further treatment is indicated.

7. Long standing or chronic Rheumatoid Disease responds slower than acute disease.

8. If a patient being treated with antiamoebics does not have a Herxheimer reaction, the patient simply does not have Rheumatoid Disease or the particular amoebae (or offending agents) are resistant to the particular antiamoebic medication being given. [There is also a possibility of lack of appropriate stomach bacteria/flora to metabolize the azoles and/or enzyme deficiencies in the patient. Ed.]

9. Herxheimer reaction signs and symptoms:
   a. General and usual: Sweating and especially night sweats, diarrhea, nausea, vomiting, headache, fever, general malaise, flushing of skin, anorexia, aching bones and "flu" symptoms resembling a serum reaction.
   b. The inflammed and affected tissues become more inflammed and tissues previously unknown to be involved become inflammed.
   c. If the urinary bladder tissues are infected, patients may develop signs of full blown cystitis.
   d. If the heart, pericardium or cardiac tissue is infected the patient may develop some paroxysmal auricular tachycardia, premature ventricular contractions or ectopic beats.
   e. If the brain or meninges are infected the patient may develop severe (temporary) depression, lethargy, generalized weakness, temporary memory loss (personal experience), irritability along with headaches.
   f. If the mouth tissues are infected, a bitter and/or metallic taste may be noted along with mild shedding or peeling of the mucosal tissues. This has also been noted in the rectal tissues.
   g. When the periosteal tissues and skeletal muscle tissues are involved, fairly severe bone pain usually accompanied by severe muscle pains and spasms may be observed, usually at night.

h. When the lungs and bronchial tissues are infected the patients may develop bronchitis symptoms and occasionally pneumonitis (resembling viral) has been observed.

From the above, one can easily see that most all of the previously observed side effects of [antiamoebics] may also be simply manifestations of the Herxheimer reaction. Therefore a clinician that is not totally knowledgeable concerning these possible signs and symptoms could easily mistake the Herxheimer reaction for possible side effects of the [antiamoebic]. Should this information not be taken into consideration, a misleading and false evaluation of any adverse experiences by various patients caused by the [antiamoebics] will be inevitable . . . the medicine could be labeled more dangerous than it actually may be, and the aggravated symptoms could be misconstrued as an intensification of the disease being treated. The information and the above facts *must be considered* in evaluating [antiamoebic] effectiveness and side effects [when treating patients].

---

[1] Herxheimer, K., *Dtsch. Mewd. Wschr.*, 1902, Vol. 28, p. 895.

[2] From Phil Gunby, *JAMA*, "Allopurinol Treatment for Protozoan Infections?" Vol. 240, No. 18, Oct. 27, 1978, p. 1941-1942; The *Limax amboeba* has a fatal flaw — a unique enzyme system that transforms allopurinol into a toxic (to the amoeba) adenine analogue, 4-amino pyrazolopyrimidine. This analogue then is incorporated into their nucleic acid, with fatal results for the protozoon.

[3] *The Causation of Rheumatoid Disease and Many Human Cancers — A New Concept in Medicine — A Précis and Addenda Including the Nature of Multiple Sclerosis*, The Rheumatoid Disease Foundation, Rt. 4, Box 137, Franklin, TN 37064, 1983, p.3.

Prior to F.M. Logsdon's (M.D.) recent death, he suggested that residual gold could be chelated from the patient by means of several EDTA treatments, using American Academy of Medical Preventics protocols. Following up the residual gold measurements by means of sera tests, he was apparently successful with several patients who thereafter responded to antiamoebics. Whether or not this will work for all, most, or many is unknown.

Chapter V
Cooperating Physicians and Scientists
How to Contact Them

The Rheumatoid Disease Foundation recommends that you take this book and its described treatment to your family physician. He/she will be given every cooperation, without charge, to help you get well.

If your family physician is unwilling to learn this treatment, then we suggest that you search your city for a physician who is open-minded. After all, it is your life — not the physician's — and you have a right to the treatment of your choice.

Try, first, those physicians who are involved with preventive medicine as they are often more open-minded than the strict allopathic physician, who wants to prescribe standard drugs according to standard practices, whether you get well or not.

And do not be afraid to try osteopathic physicians, the D.O. after their names being just as significant as an M.D.

If all else fails, then you may write to *The Rheumatoid Disease Foundation*, Rt. 4, Box 137, Franklin, TN, 37064, [(615) 646-1030] for a current list of physicians who've agreed to use these procedures.

There are many physicians scattered across the United States who use similar or equivalent procedures. How many are to be found in other countries is unknown, but *The Rheumatoid Disease Foundation* will refer where it can.

A list of physicians who've agreed to use *The Rheumatoid Disease Foundation's* treatment protocol — as of the printing date of this edition — may be found in the rear of this book.

Table of Medicines

Robert Bingham, M.D., Jack M. Blount, M.D., Archimedes A. Concon, M.D., John R.A. Simoons, Ph.D., and Professor Roger Wyburn-Mason have kindly included the following table of medicines for physicians and other readers. All but one are anti-free-living amoebic drugs, the prednisone being given *temporarily* to counter the Jarisch-Herxheimer reaction if the physician and patient desire:

Generic Name	Chemical Compound Group	Brand Name	Manufacturer
allopurinol	pyrimidine	Zyloprim®	Burroughs-Wellcome
clotrimazole*	imidazole	Mycelex®	Dome
clotrimazole*	imidazole	Lotrimin®	Delbay
diiodohydro-xyquinon	oxyquinoline	Yodoxin®	Vitarine
furazolidone	nitrofuran	Furoxone®	Eaton
metronidazole	nitroimidazole	Flagyl®	Searle
nimorazole**	nitroimidazole	Emtryl®	Salsbury
nimorazole**	nitroimidazole	Naxogin®	Erba
ornidazole**	nitroimidazole	Tiberal®	Roche
prednisone***	glucocorticoids	Deltasone®	Upjohn
rifampin	rifamycin B	Rifadin®	Dow
rifampicin	rifamycin B	Rimactane®	Ciba
tinidazole**	nitroimidazole	Fasigyn®	Pfizer
potassium para amino benzoate	vitamin B	POTABA®	Glenwood

* Available in USA only as vaginal tablets and cream.
** Not yet released by FDA for use in USA. (Tinidazole, for example, is available in Australia as Fasigyn® 500; but known as Tinidex® in Mexico without prescription)
***Prednisone is not an antiamoebic.

Tony Chapdelaine, working under Dr. Jack Neff (proto-zoologist) at Vanderbilt University, conducted extensive *in vitro* chemosensitivity tests on *Acanthamoeba culbertsoni*, *Acanthamoeba castellanni*, and *Naegleri gruberi*, finding a great variation in response to the drugs listed above, and others not listed. This variation begins to explain why some will respond immediately to treatment, while others must go through a course of several antiamoebics before acquiring a Herxheimer, and subsequent health. One medicine will kill one limax amoeba, but not another, will encyst one, but ignore another, . . . Considering that there are more than 300 different species and strains within the above two classifications, each with a different sensitivity to various chemicals, one begins to understand the variable human responses to antiamoebics.

If the amoeba is killed *in vitro*, it is likely to be killed *in vivo*. But if it is not killed *in vitro*, it may or may not be killed *in vivo*.

A classic example, is metronidazole, which does not affect any of the above species *in vitro*. It must be, therefore, that one or both of the two metabolites (both azoles) of metronidazole — (1-acetic-2-methyl-5-nitroimidazole) and (1-[2-hydroxyethyl]-2-hydroxymethyl-5-nitroimidazole) — kill the organisms *in vivo*. Possibly the small number who do not respond to metronidazole (when given protocol quantities) do not have the appropriate microflora that are necessary for producing the two active metabolites. If this is true, then physicians should consider supplementing their patient's treatment with the restoration of the necessary intestinal bacteria.

Diiodohydroxyquinon (Iodoquinol or Yodoxin®), a recent addition by Robert Bingham, M.D., was found to kill Naegleria, but not Acanthamoeba.

Clotrimazole, on the other hand, was effective in killing both genus *in vitro*, and is known to be effective *in vivo*, thus the reason for starting *Rheumatoid Disease Foundation* double-blind studies with clotrimazole.

Consider also that the *Limax amoeba*, like bacterial pathogens, is capable of losing sensitivity to one antiamoebic, and therefore each physician must consider the prospect of switching from one antiamoebic to another, especially for those who prove to be especially sensitive to the amoeba (or its products), and especially when considering the six-month anti-reinfection treatment.

Some physicians do not believe that prednisone should be used to mask the Jarisch-Herxheimer reaction, that it is better to discontinue treatment until the "allergy" reaction dies down, and then to begin antiamoebic treatment again.

Keep in mind that while physicians' experiences and opinions may vary, results are what's important!

A Simple Plea to Sincere Physicians

On Behalf of all Board Members

of *The Rheumatoid Disease Foundation*

by

GUS J. PROSCH, JR., M.D.

"If you are sincere and truly desire to relieve the agony and suffering of your arthritic patients, I beg of you to give the previously recommended treatments a trial on your rheumatoid and osteoarthritis patients. I promise you that you will receive far superior results in relieving your patients' pain, suffering and disability than anything you have ever used before. You will be treating the cause of the rheumatoid disease and not simply the symptoms. You can now offer these severely neglected patients far more than a simple 'hope' of finding relief which conventional methods of treatment cannot even offer. You will be offering them total relief which will literally change the entire lives of these patients and their families. You will never find the satisfaction and pleasure of helping your fellowman any greater than by using these techniques to treat arthritic sufferers. You will completely and thoroughly understand what I mean when certain patients come to you in a wheelchair and, after receiving your treatment and injections by the above recommended techniques, they refuse to use the wheelchair to leave your office.

"What joy! What contentment! What satisfaction!

"Good luck and God be with you!!!"

Chapter VI
Professor Wyburn-Mason's Theory of Protozoal Cause of Many Hitherto Unrelated Diseases

The Prevailing Medical Theory

Are you surprised that a simple thing, like an amoeba, is the basis, the primary cause of all your "incurable" rheumatic disease problems?

The author was, so much so that he visited Vanderbilt University Medical Library to consult with two current books of internal medicine. The following is quoted:

> **Internal medicine book 1**[1]: "On the basis of current evidence, it is more likely that rheumatoid factors are products of the host response to a more primary event. The nature of this postulated primary event is still unknown, but there is renewed interest in an old concept that microbial disease may underlie the development of rheumatoid arthritis."

> **Internal medicine book 2**[2]: "The etiologic factor(s) [causes] that set into motion the above immunological events is not known. An infectious agent, viral or bacterial, may well initiate the immunologic and subsequent inflammatory process in rheumatoid arthritis, but this hypothesis needs experimental proof."

Wyburn-Mason's Findings

Professor Roger Wyburn-Mason's 479 page book *The Causation of Rheumatoid Disease and Many Human Cancers — A New Concept In Medicine* (1978) and his *Addenda* (1983), upon which this book is based, are textbooks written for medical doctors and researchers in micro-biology, and cannot be read easily without a medical dictionary.

Wyburn-Mason's proofs, arguments, and case-histories are exceedingly well done, and lead the reader to but one conclusion: Protozoa that have been with man since his earliest evolution are still with him, and, like the bacterial theory of the origin of various diseases, these same amoebae can be cited as being the primary cause of many otherwise and hitherto unexplained diseases.

31

Indeed, since arthritic deformities are found in fossilized bones of animals that preceded man's evolution, his *Homo sapiens* structure, it must follow that this protozoon or one of a similar genus followed man's every evolutionary step.

State of Art in Medicine

By way of placing what follows in context, the author would take the liberty of itemizing some fundamental principles that the reader should consider:

1. Clinical applications in medicine always lag behind research, sometimes by as much as a generation or more. The U.S. Food and Drug Administration tightly — sometimes too conservatively — controls the use of various drugs for experimental purposes, thus inhibiting your family physician from taking advantage of early work done by others, often overseas. State medical boards, rightly or wrongly, inhibit medical practices not approved by peer review.

2. The increase in malpractice suits against physicians has brought about an almost sterile inclination to practice any kind of medicine except that which is "acceptable" by text-book peer review. If the text-book says that something cannot be cured, and that one should, however, treat symptoms, then that is what your doctor will tell his patient, and what he will do, respectively. It keeps *him* out of trouble, although it has virtually no chance of curing you.

3. The theory of protozoa as sources of disease in the human body has only recently been opened by the general medical profession, and the theory has only now been fully developed by the research of Professor Wyburn-Mason and shown in the above named book.

4. There is already a well-developed theory of *bacteria* as primary source of disease, a well-developed theory of *fungus* and *yeasts* as cause of disease, a growing development of *viral* cause of disease, a new theory of *viroids* and *prions* (stripped-down virus), and a very sporadically developed theory of *protozoon* (amoeboid) cause of disease, until now.

5. Consider the original, historical impact of the theory of

bacteria as primary source of disease. Once you get the idea that there are many different species and strains of bacteria and that when they invade humans they each affect different systems and organs in different ways, one can begin to understand the parallel protozoal theory. Broad-spectrum antibiotics can be used interchangeably against microbial caused diseases thereby demonstrating many different symptoms and bringing about a cure of each. So it is with the protozoon theory of disease. There are over 300 species of amoebae identified to date, some of which are pathogenic, and certain broad-spectrum anti-protozoal medicines will knock them out, no matter what the ultimate symptoms may appear to be, and no matter how those symptoms are currently classified in medical literature. Remember, *symptoms classifications are only that, not descriptions of primary causes!*

6. According to Professor Roger Wyburn-Mason's work, there are certain protozoa that are called *Limax* (*Limax amoeba*: meaning slug-like amoeba) that are found in virtually all human and animal tissue from birth onward. Similar to the ever-present bacterias, these *Limax amoebae* may be pathogenic and may affect different parts of the human body in different ways, depending upon their species, your genetic heritage, and upon which systems or organs they invade. Their hostile invasions are apparently triggered off within the body in the same manner and for the same reasons that multiplication of hostile bacteria begins.

7. These *Limax amoebae* were not found in many diseases previously because (a) it was thought to take special staining techniques to find them, (b) when they are found they are often mistaken for the body's own macrophages or poorly stained leucocytes, (c) even when animals are inoculated with them and similar diseases produced in the animals, the amoebae are difficult to find in the lesions, although *the live protozoa can be separated from tissue by special techniques.*

8. In Chapter IV of Professor Wyburn-Mason's book (pages 120-1) it is stated that the *Limax amoebae* were isolated from:

a. all the tissues of all cases of collagen and auto-immune diseases examined, including cases of rheumatoid arthritis, systemic lupus erythematosus (disease producing symptoms on skin), lymphocytic thyroid lesions (infection of thyroid), salivary glands affected by Sjögren's syndrome (inflammation of parotid glands; arthritis; dryness of mouth from lack of secretion) etc. In these cases it was found not only in the region of the affected joints, muscles, thyroid and salivary glands, but also in the spleen, lymph nodes and central nervous system, and, in fact, in all apparently normal tissues.

b. all body tissues in all cases of human leukaemia (disease of blood-forming organs) and lymphoma (disease of lymphoid tissue) examined.

c. all of a large number of human and animal malignant tumors examined, when it occurred in large numbers in the tumor itself, but in lesser numbers in all the unaffected tissues of the body.

d. all aborted material exhibiting congenital growth anomalies examined and in many normal placentae.

e. hypertrophied tonsils and adenoids removed at operation.

f. the normal tissues in many healthy subjects killed in accidents.

g. human and mammalian faecal material.

h. uncooked beef, mutton, pork, and eggs and unsterilized milk.

i. some specimens of surface soil.

j. certain plant tumors growing at the site where the stem passes through the soil.

9. The *Limax amoeba* was not found in laboratory mice and rat cancers.

Primary Source of Rheumatic Diseases

The protozoon theory as the primary source of rheumatoid diseases is simply this:

1. The *Limax* amoebae are found virtually everywhere in the world, and inhabit virtually all animal bodies, including man's. Encysted forms (spheres filled with reproductive material and holes through which this can escape) are taken into the body through air, water and food and adult forms are found in the feces of most animals, including man. We

arc constantly infected and re-infected with both pathogenic (disease producing) and nonpathogenic forms. *Such protozoa form part of our natural environment* and are quite unlike and unrelated to those forms of parasitic amoebae which cause amoebic dysentery in man.

2. In certain individuals stress, or the taking into their body of certain pathogenic species of amoebae, causes the body tissues containing the organisms to react to their presence and become inflamed, providing the organism is pathogenic and the patient's individual cells contain certain genes which make them react to the presence in the tissues of these organisms, where its products are recognized as antigens[3] by our bodily defenses. This reaction to the presence of the organism is genetically controlled, so the disease may run in families.

3. The reaction to the presence of these foreign and pathogenic organisms consists of the proliferation of certain cells called lymphocytes and their derivative plasma cells, which produce antibodies against the antigens of the organism. These antibodies are present in the blood plasma forming immunoglobulins. Both the blood cells and chemicals attempt to destroy the foreign bodies and in so doing fail to discriminate between them and many normal tissues in the body. As Dr. Jack M. Blount explains, "like innocent bystanders they get hit by bullets aimed at an invader, our own immune system attacks both the invader and our own tissues, thus the name 'autoimmune disease'." However, though these blood changes are undoubtedly present, no one until now has been able to find their cause, though it has frequently been suggested that they are due to some unknown infection. These inflammatory changes may involve any tissue in the body.

4. Many other micro and macro events abound, but simply stated, it appears as though the inflammatory changes and destruction of joints is partially due to the presence of the amoeba and partially due to the lymphocytes and result in immunoglobulin changes in the blood. This is true of all the tissues of the body.

5. Two physicians have confirmed Professor Roger Wyburn-Mason's findings of protozoa in the tissues[4]; and also by

England's Air Vice Marshall Stamm[5]; and also by Raymond Cursons[6], New Zealand, that the sera of all living humans and even the cord blood, contains antibodies against free-living amoebae, whether pathogenic or non-pathogenic, indicating that everybody is infected by these protozoa. Craig and Faust[7] state that unspecified types of amoebae have been isolated from every tissue in the body, while Dobell C.[8] states "there is hardly an organ in the body from which somebody has not obtained amoebae." Dr. Bradley, a microbiologist, has positively identified antibodies against *Naegleria fowleri* in the blood of his patients[9]!

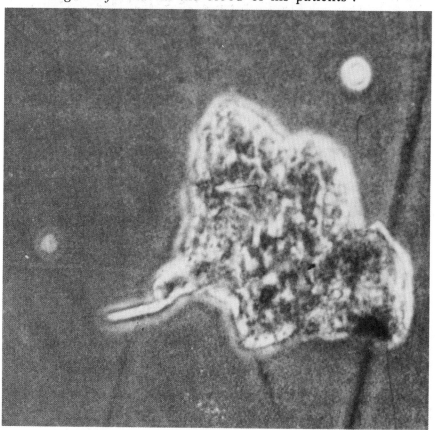

Photograph of a Limax *amoeba which emigrated from the malignant tissue in a case of carcinoma of the bronchus (unstained). (X1500). Note single spike-like pseudopodium, typical of many species of Naegleria*.*

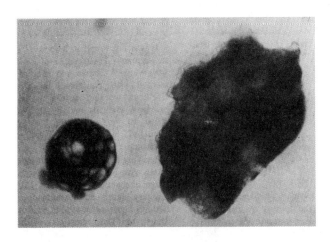

A cyst of Limax amoeba *beside a trophozoite heavily pigmented as recovered from human malignant tissue. The pigmentation is presumably due to phagocytosis of debris from the minced-up tumor tissue (unstained) (X2000)*. [Compare with Figure 2 in Jager and Stamm (1972).]*

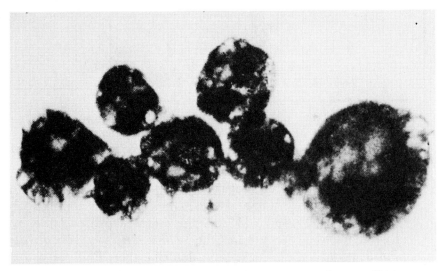

Cysts of Limax amoeba *formed after migration from malignant tumors under the influence of thermotropism (unstained). Shows simultaneous cyst formation from a cluster of trophozoites (X950)*.*

*Wyburn-Mason, Roger, *The Causation of Rheumatoid Disease and Many Human Cancers — A New Concept in Medicine*, Iji Publishing Co., Tokyo, Japan, 1978, p 122. (Note: This book is now out of print, but Jack M. Blount, Jr., M.D. has furnished a number of copies to various medical school and hospital libraries.)

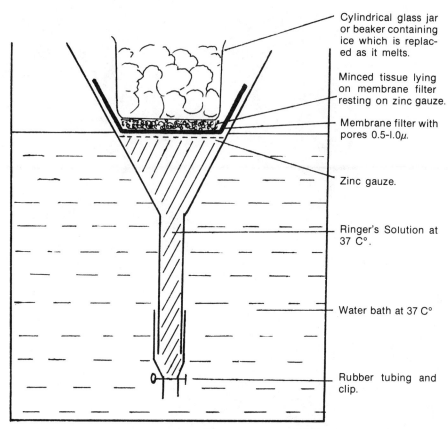

Drawing of apparatus used to enable migration of organism to take place *under thermotropic influences. Note: do no use copper screen as the copper ion will kill the amoebae. (Used by courtesy Professor Roger Wyburn-Mason).*

6. Most amazing, after Roger Wyburn-Mason's discovery of the organism in human tissues, there is found a published report in 1922[10] and 1924 by the eminent protozoologists, Kofoid and Swezy, in the *University of California Publications of Zoology*, who describe their findings in the bone marrow of cases of rheumatoid arthritis and the lymph nodes of Hodgkin's disease. (**Dr. Roger Wyburn-Mason's work was confirmed 50 years earlier!**). The two protozoologists suggested an aetiological relationship to the arthritic process, but they published this in a zoological journal, so that their findings never received the interest they deserved. (In 1969, Dr. S.L. Warren and Dr. Leonard

Marmor[1] reported finding an agent in tissue drawn from patients with rheumatoid arthritis which could be transmitted to mice producing inflammatory changes. Since then the substance [which appears to be an infectious nucleic acid precipitate] has been found in synovial tissues removed from the joints of patients with classical symptoms of advanced acute rheumatoid arthritis. It appears to be present during the early and active stages of arthritis when the disease is spreading from joint to joint. The limax amoeba is found in the micro-circulation. Some researchers suspect that the limax amoeba are the *carriers* of the rheumatoid arthritis ribonucleic acid infective agent.)

7. But even without confirmation of the limax amoeba the fact that antiprotozoal medicines bring about the Jarisch-Herxheimer reaction in suffering arthritics, and healthy patients do not react in like manner, proves the presence in the lesions of rheumatoid arthritis of an amoeba[12].

8. The organisms have been demonstrated in tissues by immunofluorescent staining of sections to which antisera to the organisms have been added [13].

9. A condition almost identical with rheumatoid arthritis may complicate amoebic dysentery, but in this case the organisms are not in the tissues, and patients do not exhibit the Herxheimer reaction with antiamoebic drugs.

10. Thus, if the protozoal theory is correct, when we seek to cut down inflammation and pain in rheumatoid arthritis with anti-inflammatory drugs (as with aspirin and aspirin substitutes), we are simply decreasing symptomatic responses, and leaving the protozoa free to continue proliferating and causing further damage.

11. Again, if the protozoal theory is correct, when we seek to knock out the immunological system (as with imuran treatment) we are simply freeing the protozoa from any check and balance, and so it can be expected to continue proliferating and causing further damage.

12. If the protozoal theory is correct, when we seek to block the interaction between antigen and anti-body (as with cortisone treatment), we are simply freeing the protozoa for further action.

13. If the protozoal theory is correct, then some weeks of the

antiprotozoal drugs should bring about immediate relief in most symptoms, especially as the body no longer finds need to react against the invader, and the immunological system can then settle down — *and this is exactly what Professor Roger Wyburn-Mason*[14] *and Dr. Jack M. Blount and other researchers have found happens.*

[1] *Fifteenth Edition of the Cecil Textbook of Medicine, Vol. I,* W.B. Saunders Co., Philadelphia 1979, p. 187.

[2] *Harrison's Principles of Internal Medicine, 9th Edition, Vol. II,* McGraw-Hill Book Co., New York, 1980, p. 1873.

[3] From "The Genetics of Antibody Diversity" by Philip Leder, *Scientific American,* Vol. 246, Number 5, May 1982, p. 102, we learn: "[Our] immune system has a virtually unlimited capacity to generate different antibodies, which recognize and bind to many millions of potential antigens, or 'nonself' molecules. . . . An antibody is an assembly of protein chains, and the structure of a protein chain is specified by a unit of genetic information: a gene. . . . Antibodies, like other proteins, are made up of the subunits called amino acids. There are 20 kinds of amino acid, which can be linked together in any combination to form a protein chain. The amino acid composition of a chain and the sequence in which the amino acids are arrayed along the chain determine how the chain folds in three dimensions and perhaps combines with other chains. . . .The amino acid composition and sequence of a protein chain are prescribed by [the] gene."

[4] James W. Overstreet III was in the Microbiology Department, Vanderbilt University, Nashville, Tennessee, USA in 1965, according to a personal letter from Professor Roger Wyburn-Mason to author. In a letter dated February 1, 1983 to Wyburn-Mason, James W. Overstreet, M.D., Ph.D., now Associate Professor of Human Anatomy and Obstetrics and Gynecology at University of California, Davis, states: "Thank you for your letter of January 22, 1983. I am the same individual who corresponded with you in 1965. At that time, I was a second year undergraduate student and the work on protozoa recovered from human tissue was my first independent research project. I thought you might be interested in my curriculum vitae since it details my subsequent professional career. As you see, I spent several years in Cambridge where my research interests became focused on the area of Reproductive Biology. Although I never pursued the work on protozoa, I believe that project and your encouragement were significant factors in my decision to pursue a career in medical research."; and Magda Uhrinova, Oncological Research institute, Bratislavia, Czechoslovakia [from Professor Roger Wyburn-Mason, who states: "Dr. Magda Uhrinova and Dr. A. Kwasnicka working together also isolated the organism in the same way as I had done and, when I visited them in 1965, they showed me photographs of beautiful examples of the organism which I understand was reported to the House Journal of the Institute in that year; I have since lost touch with them."]

[5] The doyen of amoebologists [personal letter from Professor Roger Wyburn-Mason who states: "Air Vice Marshall Stamm has long ago retired. He worked at the Institute of Amoebology which was then part of the Royal Free Hospital, London. Since his retirement the Institute has closed and this work is largely taken over by the London School of Hygiene and Tropical Medicine. I sent a number of slides to Air Vice Marshall Stamm apparently containing no amoebae visible by ordinary stains, but out of which I had obtained them. The slides consisted of tissue taken from the enlarged salivary glands in cases of rheumatoid disease, Hodgkin's disease, knee joint tissue and muscle taken from cases of rheumatoid disease and in addition various cancers. I asked him to test them by immunological staining using antibodies to various species of *Naegleria amoebae* for evidence of amoebae and in a number of phone calls and a letter he was highly

enthusiastic and had confirmed by his very selective method of staining that certain cells in the tissues gave the typical stains for *Naeglerian* though in ordinary circumstances they did not resemble them, but looked like macrophages. He did not, however, publish his findings as those were going to be included in my book. His findings are those cited by me in my book and were taken from his letter."]

6 Cursons, R.T.M., T.J. Brown and E.A. Keys *Lancet*, 1977, ii, 875.

7 Craig and Faust, *Clinical Parasitology*, 6th ed. Henry Kimpton,London, 1957, p. 211.

8 Dobell C., *The Amoebae Living in Man*, John Bell Sons and Dainelsson, London, 1919, p. 90.

9 Personal correspondence from John R.A. Simoons, Ph.D. to Dr. J.M. Blount, November 5, 1981.

10 Kofoid, C.A.; Swezy, O., "Amebiasis of the Bones", *J. Amer. Med. Ass.*, 78:1602-1604, 1922a; also "Mitosis in Endamoeba Dysenteriae in the Bone Marrow in Arthritis Deformans", *Univ. Calif. Publ. Zool.* 20:301-307, 1922b; also "On the Occurrence of Endamoeba Dysenteriae in the Bone Lesions of Arthritis Deformans", *Calif. State J. Med.* 20:59; 1922c. Kofoid, C.A.; Boyers, L.M.; Swezy, O. "Endamoeba Dysenteriae in the Lymph Glands of Man in Hodgkin's Disease", *Univ. Calif. Publ. Zool.* 20:309-312; 1922a; also "Occurrence of Endamoeba Dysenteriae in the Lesions of Hodgkin's Disease", *J. Amer. Med. Ass.* 78:1604-1607; 1922b; and Kofoid, C.A.; Swezy, O.; Boyers, L.M., "The Coexistence of Hodgkin's Disease and Amoebiasis", *J. Amer. Med. Ass.*, 78:1602-1604, 1922; [from Professor Roger Wyburn-Mason: Also "later publication in 1925 in the *Univ. Calif. Publ. Zool.* where they changed the name of the organism to that of *Vahlkampfia*, which is free-living amoeba. The organism that they found in the bone marrow differed from normal cells in that it contained only 6 chromosomes as compared with the normal 46 of humans and its method of mitosis (multiplying) and possessed one pseudopodium which is identical with the organism as found by" Professor Wyburn-Mason].

11 *Arthritis News Today*, Vol. 1, No. 10, "Progress on the Cause and Treatment of Rheumatoid Arthritis," P.O. Box 730, Yorba Linda, California 92686, July 1979, pp. 1-2.

12 P.K. Pybus SA *Mediese Tydskrif*, "Metronidazole in Rheumatoid Arthritis," Februarie 20, 1982, p. 261-262.

13 According to one of Professor Roger Wyburn-Mason's latest communications, "Dr. P.K. Pybus and Dr. A.E. Davis, both of South Africa, have recently informed of a very simple method of isolating the organism and the cysts from the effusion fluids of actively inflamed rheumatoid knee joints. Using a sterile needle and syringe they withdrew all the fluid from inflamed knees and put this into a sterile screwtop bottle. They allowed this to stand and cool for a few hours and then examined the deposit. In all cases the deposits contained groups of typical free-living amoebic cysts identical in appearance with those in Figure 1 of the article by Jager and Stamm (*Lancet* 1972, ii, 1943) featuring the cysts of an organism of the Naegerial genus. The size, the fenestrated holes allowing the cytoplasm of the cysts to escape and the varying colouration of the cysts from dark brown to light brown, dark blue to light blue, are typical of the same cysts photographed by the present author as being found with their trophozoites in rheumatoid disease and cancers and photographed at Figure 7, page 123 in the original monograph. The variation in colour found by both Pybus and Davis and the author caused the latter to christen the organism, amoeba chromatosa (coloured amoeba). In addition Pybus and Davis sometimes found the motile amoebae apparently attempting ingestion of red blood cells and sometimes in the process of encystment. These workers remarked that these objects one would normally dismiss as cell de'bris or 'gubbins', but in view of their features they are undoubtedly small amoebae."

14 Professor Roger Wyburn-Mason had spent 27 years in the field of protozoology, pharmacology and rheumatology.

"Of course one does meet brilliant men but they are isolated. The fashion nowadays is all for groups and societies of every sort. It is always a sign of mediocrity in people when they herd together . . . . The truth is only sought by individuals, and they break with those who do not love it enough . . . ." — Dr. Zhivago *by Boris Pasternak.*

ROGER WYBURN-MASON

Letter received, June 1983

I have been thinking over the significance of the discovery of the cause and cure of rheumatoid disease in all parts of the world.

To begin with the treatment and cure of the early disease prevents patients becoming chair-bound and bed-ridden and eventually taking up beds in hospitals for the physically handicapped, which in your country and my own and in all countries of the civilized world is an enormous drain on financial resources.

In addition while the patient is gradually developing the disease over the course of years he has with the so-called orthodox treatment long periods off work in which he is paid for by the state either at home or in hospital absorbing enormous amounts of expensive anti-inflammatory or immunodepressant drugs very often paid for by the state and requiring medical and nursing attention throughout the active period of the diseases. In spite of this the disease makes its inevitable painful progress.

In children the disease causes painful deformity often treated with cortisone derivatives which stunt growth and do not kill the cause of the disease. They end in homes for the incurable provided by the state.

From these observations it is obvious that treatment of RD by anti-free-living amoebic drugs will result in the saving of enormous amounts of money by the state in providing hospital accomodation, doctors, nurses, drugs and apparatus, while if the patient is not hospitalized he remains ill at home where he has to be nursed and doctored and the Government pay his unemployment benefit.

The discovery of the cause of the disease and its cure will have an important financial bearing on the state and country providing all the above mentioned aids in the commonest disease afflicting mankind and the one causing more suffering and disability than any other.

Within ten years the disease could probably be eliminated from civilized countries setting free enormous amounts of money to be used for other purposes.

Chapter VII
Amazing Implications of the Protozoon Discovery

Broad-spectrum Antibiotics

As has been already stated, when the germ theory of disease was at last accepted, many disease symptoms could be seen to respond to similar or identical medicines. In later years, particularly stemming from the development of sulpha-like and penicillin-like drugs, we have seen many apparently dissimilar diseases respond to identical drugs, now called *broad-spectrum* medicines because of their ability to inhibit or kill a variety of species or genus within species of bacteria.

Broad-spectrum Antiamoebics

Professor Roger Wyburn-Mason asserts in his massive study that the same is true regarding protozoa as a primary cause of other diseases.

Isolation of the Amoeba

He was able to recover the free-living amoebae (to be distinguished from parasitic amoebae) from human tissues in certain conditions by using the property of these organisms to migrate from cold to body tissues to fluid at body temperature (37° C). When this is done, the organisms can be grown in the laboratory and various substances can be tested on them to see which kill them. Among the latter are drugs containing the 5-nitroimidazole nucleus of which one is the metronidazole or Flagyl®, but numerous others exist, such as allopurinol. In addition furazolidone, clotrimazole, and other substances are effective in killing the organisms, but are unavailable in USA.

Collagen Diseases

Closely related to rheumatoid arthritis are the so-called collagen diseases. These include systemic lupus erythematosus (SLE), dermato-(poly-) myositis, scleroderma (systemic sclerosis) and polyarteritis nodosa, and every gradation to or combination of these various conditions with rheumatoid arthritis exists and these diseases may be associated with internal manifestations of the same process as affects the joints.

In SLE the presence of the causative organism in the body produces changes in the proteins of the blood which may deposit in the walls of blood vessels which then cut off the blood supply to parts of the brain or kidney especially. When these changes have occurred treatment with antiamoebics cannot cure the disease completely, but can halt its progress. The same applies to advanced cases of rheumatoid disease, though the cause of the disease may be killed and damaged joints may be treated by other means such as surgical or chelation therapy.

The other diseases mentioned above can be cured in early cases in the same way as rheumatoid arthritis.

Some cases of rheumatoid arthritis or any of the collagen diseases may be associated with mild diabetes or the rare muscular disease known as myasthenia gravis.

Myasthenia gravis appears to be due to liberation from infecting amoebae of substances which combine with the chemical substances normally liberated at the nerve endings in muscles thus inactivating and preventing muscle contraction and producing weakness.

Diabetes is not due to failure of the cells of the pancreas to produce sufficient insulin to enable the muscle and liver cells to store sugar in them. This was the theory until some years ago when a United States Professor[1] received the Nobel Prize for medicine by showing that in diabetes the pancreas produces either normal or excessive amounts of insulin in diabetics.

Diabetes is, in fact, due to inactivation of the normally formed insulin by some substance in the body. If a patient suffering from diabetes is treated with the antiamoebic drugs, the mild diabetes will disappear unless the patient becomes reinfected with the organism. Until the recovery of the free-living amoebae from the tissues of cases of rheumatoid disease the generally held idea was that the disease was due to a chronic antigenic stimulation though the source of this antigen was unknown. We now know that the amoeba is the source of this antigen which induces the production by lymphocytes and plasma cells of antibodies in the blood.

Susceptibility

The presence in all bodies, including the newborn, of the organisms (transmitted across the placenta to the foetus) may produce no damage or signs of its presence unless the species is of a pathogenic type and even then it may not produce disease in humans unless the cells of the human's body possess certain genes which are inherited from the parents which enable them to become inflamed in the presence of the organisms. In this way whole families may be affected by rheumatoid disease.

44

Rheumatoid disease may affect any tissue in the body and produce what are known as precancerous lesions, i.e. changes in tissues which may develop into cancer.

Treatment with antiamoebics can cure those precancerous lesions and the tendency for them to become cancerous, but this requires a course of treatment repeated perhaps yearly or so. If no reaction to the antiamoebic medicines occurs, then the individual is free of pathogenic infection. If a reaction does occur, the individual is infected and even if there is no evidence of active rheumatoid disease, such an individual may have internal changes due to the organism, which may develop into cancer.

The Rheumatoid Disease Foundation recommends that allopurinol be taken at six month intervals to prevent reinfections. Whenever the patient appears highly susceptible, and/or the geographical region appears to offer maximum opportunities for reinfection, antiamoebics could be taken every two months. Public water systems, swimming pools, dust farming, meat handling . . . are often excellent sources of reinfection.

The copper ion seems to be rather deadly to the amoebae but chlorine, as used for purifying our drinking water, is not.

William Catterall, Sc.D., recommends a copper algicide for swimming pools; and while the limax amoebae are very sensitive to small amounts of copper ion — such as placing a copper wire in refrigerator drinking water — he cautions against intake of too much copper, as this can upset the mineral ratios or even be dangerous.

Small doses of antiamoebics taken at semi-annual intervals may also prevent mild but obvious joint aches and pains, a sign that fluid movement is being inhibited and also an early sign of rheumatoid arthritis. If allopurinol is taken, then 3 tablets (300 mgm) a day each day for seven days should be sufficient to remove reinfections, and the resulting Herxheimer, if any, will probably be much less than the first full treatment; if a different antiamoebic is used, then a different number of tablets may be required.

In both cases, the number of tablets will also depend upon body weight. Obviously children, or people of above average or below average weight, should be given differing dosages, usually determined in terms of 20# increments.

Regular doses will avoid cancerous change in some cases. Quite apart from the prospect of being able to prevent the appalling suffering and deformities of long-standing cases of rheumatoid arthritis and its internal lesions, one can cure the disease in children and eventually the prospect of wiping out probably the commonest disease in the world opens up.

In addition to this, there is the possibility of preventing the development of many cancers by curing the pre-malignant diseases, which are part of rheumatoid arthritis. As stated, the presence in the body of the organisms with their antigens stimulates the appropriate cells (lymphocytes and plasma cells) found in the bone marrow to produce antibodies against these cells. If long continued, the bone marrow cells proliferate and change into cancerous cells called myeloma or lymphoma, so that the chronic infection with the amoebae is a very important cause of cancer. These growths can be prevented by taking yearly treatment with antiamoebic drugs only some of which are available in the United States, but all of which are harmless, as opposed to the present anti-inflammatory drugs and cortisone.

Present Rheumatology Practices Unscientific[2]

From the discovery that rheumatoid arthritis is due to an organism around the lesions certain practices commonly found in rheumatology are seen to be unscientific:

Firstly, *all present anti-inflammatory drugs, gold salts and penicillamine have side effects which may be so dangerous as to kill the patient either by damage to the bone marrow, and thus failure to produce the essential blood corpuscles, damage to the kidney resulting in kidney failure, or to the skin which may peel off the whole body giving rise to severe and uncontrollable infection resulting in death, as in the case of the film actress Rosalind Russell.* **This group of drugs has never *cured* a patient.** *Whereas the drugs used to kill the amoeba have all been used for twenty or more years without causing ill effects.* ***These antiamoebic medicines are frequently successful in completely curing the disease.*** Like bacteria, different amoebae show different susceptibilities to different antiamoebic drugs. It may be necessary to switch from one to another to obtain the best results. (Alcohol should not be taken during treatment.)

Secondly massage and exercising affected joints are guaranteed to spread the organism about and make the condition worse. Affected joints should be rested and cooled with water (not ice) and never massaged.

It is quite clear from the amazing list covered by Professor Wyburn-Mason's work, that he has opened a realm of medical applications that is strikingly unusual to say the least[3]. Causes for some diseases are unknown, some are classified as hereditary, and some are flatly blamed on viral infections, while others are diseases of behavior or thought. Yet anti-protozoon drugs seem to affect cures, with exceptions noted in Wyburn-Mason's book (such as arthritis caused by bacteria or physical shock, et. al.)

Keep in mind that symptom descriptions are only that, *descriptions*, and not necessarily indicative of the causes. When the *Limax amoeba* attacks one kind of tissue, and depending upon your particular (inherited) body chemistry, you may have a set of symptoms totally different than would another from the same amoeba.

Since application of antiamoebic drugs is novel in the treatment of most of the diseases listed, you should work with your family

---

[1] Rosalyn S. Yalow, 1977, who shared one half the prize with two others, Roger C.L. Guillemin and Andrew V. Schally.

[2] For analysis of the unscientific nature of present rheumatology practices, see *Clinics in Rheumatic Diseases*, December 1983, W.B. Saunders, Ltd., West Washington Square, Philadelphia, PA 19105. Especially read the chapters on gold shots and pencillamine, and the lack of scientific basis, as described by leading rheumatologists.

[3] In the second edition, Crohn's disease was added to the list below by Dr. Gus J. Prosch; trigeminal neuralgia and multiple sclerosis has been added by further research of Roger Wyburn-Mason, with precautionary statements given on applying anti-amoebics to multiple sclerosis footnoted below the list. [See his *Addenda, The Causation of Rheumatoid Disease and Many Human Cancers — A New Concept in Medicine: A Précis and Addenda, Including the Nature of Multiple Sclerosis*, The Rheumatoid Disease Foundation, Box 137, Franklin, TN 37064, $7.50 plus $1.00 handling.]

Dr. Jack M. Blount, states that manifestations of infection vary with the anatomy involved, the genetic composition of tissue affected, and the nature of the infestation. To your family doctor he says, "Compare to *Treponema pallidum* (Syphilis spirochete) symptoms — may involve any organ or tissue . . . relapses frequent, may exist without symptoms for years."

Roger Wyburn-Mason, in his *Addenda*, [p. 7] adds the following: "AI lymphocytic and humoral reactions are thus not the primary disturbance in RD and AI diseases, but are the response to the tissue damage. The whole syndrome resembles syphilis. Waldenström (1963) and others state that 'if the spirocheate had not been discovered, syphilis could be taken to be the ideal model of an AI disease. The variety of tissue reaction antibodies, the widespread lymphocytic tissue damage and the vasculitis are characteristic features.' RD closely resembles the rheumatoic manifestations in leprosy (*Lancet* Editorial 1981), which may present with an acute arthritis affecting one or a number of joints, polymyositis, skin lesions, fever, raised ESR, etc. with increase in circulating gamma-globulins and positive serological tests for autoantibodies, RF and ANF, as in RD. This is an immune complex syndrome with antigen provided by disintegrating *M. leprae*. The reaction may be precipitated by anti-leprosy drugs, a reaction known as Lucio's phenomenon, **which is identical with the Herxheimer reaction**." [Emphasis author's]

47

physician in seeking treatment, or, failing that, contact any of the medical doctors already working with this treatment.

Tissues affected are:
Arteries: Periarteritis
Bone: Paget's Disease, cysts, myelomas
Brain and Cord: Tremors, seizures
Bronchi: Bronchitis, intrinsic asthma
Cardiac: Dysrhythmias, myocardial disease, pericardial disease
Cecum: Appendicitis, mesenteric adenitis
Colon: Ulcerative colitis
Endocrine: Thyroid, parathyroid, thymus, pituitary, adrenal, gonads
Esophagus and Stomach: Atropic mucosa (pernicious anemia), webs
Eyes: Iridocyclitis, exophthalmias
Fasical Planes: Bursitis
Female Genitals: Ovarian cysts, fibroids, salpingitis-sterility, tubal pregnancies
Functional CNS: Neuroses, psychoses, senility
Hemopoetic: Systemic lupus erythematosus, polycythemia, purpura
Joints: Arthritis
Kidneys: Pyelonephritis, calculi
Liver: Hepatitis, cholangitis, gallbladder disease
Lower Small Gut: Regional enteritis, Crohn's disease
Lungs: Alveolitis
Lymphatics: Lymphomas, splenomegaly
Meninges: Headache, meningomas
Muscles: Myositis
Nerves*: Trigeminal neuralgia*, [**multiple sclerosis***]
Nose and Throat: Rhinitis, eustachian salpingitis, enlarged tonsils, & adenoids, etc.
Ovum: Fetal deformities, abortions
Pancreas: Pancreatitis, maturity diabetes, noninsulin dependent diabetes
Salivary & Tear Glands: SICCA syndrome
Skin: Psoriasis, alopecia, erythemas, urticaria
Spine: Degenerated discs, low back syndrome
Tendons: Tendonitis, ganglion
Upper Gut: Coealic disease

Important Note

* From *Addenda* [Roger Wyburn-Mason, p. 26, 28-29]: ". . . The makers of 5-nitroimididazole drugs warn against administration to patients suffering from neurological disease, but none of them on close enquiry can give the reason for this warning. . . . MS is due to the presence in the CNS [central nervous system] of pathogenic free-living amoebae in a sensitive subject as evidenced by the tissue antigens and that sudden destruction of the organisms by anti-free living amoebic substances can cause a sudden and violent exaggeration of symptoms due to the action of drugs on the organisms within the CNS. Can such drugs be used in the treatment of MS without running the risk of exaggeration of symptoms? . . . [It is possible that] antiamoebic drugs [that do not produce] an Herxheimer reaction might . . . be used to prevent the progress of MS by killing the causative agent and preventing the formation of new plaques. . . . "

Chapter VIII
Case Histories

(Based on Professor Roger Wyburn-Mason, Surrey, England, in which two new anti-protozoon compounds furazolidone *and* allopurinol *were used in the treatment of rheumatoid arthritis. These compounds have been safely in use for many years for other diseases.)*

Introduction

Furazolidone is an antibacterial and antiprotozoon drug effective against a wide range of common enteric infections, both bacterial and protozoon, such as *Giardia lamblia* and *Entamoeba histolytica*.

It was found that in vitro a dilute solution rapidly killed the organisms in a culture of the free-living amoebae isolated from the tissues of rheumatoid and related diseases being equally or more potent in this respect to the 5-nitroimidazoles.

Allopurinol has been reported as being effective treatment of the protozoon diseases Leishmaniasis and Trypanosomiasis and it shows promising results in the treatment of *Trypanosoma cruzi* infections and diseases due to other haemoflagellates[1].

Free-living amoebae of the genus *Naegleria* assume a flagellate form in distilled water and [Wyburn-Mason] found that in vitro the drug killed the cells of a culture of amoebae obtained from the tissues of patients with rheumatoid disease in very dilute solution, being equally or more effective in this respect than the 5-nitroimidazoles.

Antiamoebic substances without anti-inflammatory properties, which kill free-living amoebae in cases of active rheumatoid disease[2] often produce an Jarisch-Herxheimer reaction, indicative of the presence of such a causative organism in this disease.

It was decided to test the effect of these safe and long-established substances (furazolidone and allopurinol) in cases of active rheumatoid disease, in view of [Wyburn-Mason's] previous findings of the curative effect of many antiamoebic substances.

When taking furazolidone patients have occasionally been reported as having nausea or headache and facial flushing if they take alcohol. Both substances tend to cause dark yellow coloration of the urine and this prevents their use in a double blind trial.

The following are the details of successive cases of active

49

rheumatoid disease treated in a rheumatology practice with furazolidone in doses of 100 mg four times a day for 7 days or with allopurinol 300 mg three times daily for 10 days.

Successive cases treated with furazolidone

Case 1: Female, aged 62 years. Family History: Mother, one brother and two sisters all suffered from rheumatoid arthritis while one brother and one sister are free of the disease. A nephew and one sister suffered from diabetes.
Past history: Her periods ceased at the age of 40 years. Ten years previously she noticed painless thickening and stiffness of all joints of the fingers and thumbs gradually increasing in degree and eleven months previously she woke up one morning with painful and swollen fingers and wrist joints, increasing in severity over the next two months. Her knees were also affected and her symptoms became so severe that she was unable to use her hands. Four months later the right knee and both elbows became painful and swollen, movements were restricted and she developed bursitis of both elbows followed by pain and restricted movements of the right shoulder. She was treated with numerous anti-inflammatory drugs, including steroid injections into the shoulder joints and olecranon bursae. Five months previous to being seen she developed bilateral carpal tunnel compression of the median nerve for which operation was undertaken successfully. X-rays showed some slight loss of disc space in the first carpometacarpal joints, but otherwise the appearances were within normal limits.
The serum RF was strongly positive. Blood sedimentation rate was 30 mm/hour. RBC was 3.9×10^{12}/dl, serum albumin 2.8, globulin 3.8 g/dl, WBC 4.8×10^9/dl, Hb 10.9 g/dl.
She was at present taking 3 Naprosyn® tablets a day with little relief. There was morning stiffness and stiffness after sitting. Examination showed marked rheumatoid deformity of hands and thumbs and of the metacarpohalangeal joints. She could not make a fist. The changes of rheumatoid arthritis with heat and swelling were present in both wrists. Restriction of the shoulders, neck and midtarsal joint movements, and some swelling of the feet was present.
She was treated with furazolidone, which produced dark yellow coloration of the urine, stiffness and swelling of the affected joints on waking, but less pain in the shoulder joints. On the fifth day the symptoms had all increased in severity with increased swelling and pain in the knees with limitation of flexion, but no free fluid. The symptoms persisted for the next week when they gradually subsided and after one month had completely disappeared. She was now able to make a fist on both sides, but there was no tenderness of any joint.
Two months after beginning treatment she had been able to give up taking Naprosyn® and all joint movements were full, free and painless. There was only minimal bony swelling in the proximal interphalangeal joints of the fingers which had been present for 10 years. Blood examination now showed ESR 10 mms/hour, RBC 5.0 $\times 10^{12}$/dl, WBC 5.6×10^4/dl, serum albumin 4.6, globulin 3.2 g/dl, Hb 14.2 g/dl. She remained well for the next eight months of observation.

Case 2: Female, aged 63 years. Family history: nil revelant.
Past history, hysterectomy for fibroids and bilateral ovarian cysts aged 49 years. Three years previously she developed pain, heat, hotness and restricted movements of the fingers, wrists, neck, elbows, shoulders, hips, knees and ankles. There was pain under the balls of the feet on weight bearing. There were posterior headaches and nocturnal sweating. In addition she had all the symptoms and signs of proven ulcerative colitis. She also had considerable weight loss though her appetite was good. She had

been treated elsewhere with Indocid®, Feldene®, Froben®, brufen, penicillamine, myocrisin, and salazoprin for diarrhoea.

Examination showed a high color in the cheeks, mildly pale mucosae, pain and swelling of the fingers and wrist joints with deformities of the wrists, left alecranon bursitis, pain and restricted movements of the shoulders making it impossible for her to feed herself or to raise her arms above 45° from the body. Both knees showed lipomata below the patella, though the movements were reasonable and full, but painful on the left side. There was slight pain on extreme movements of the left ankle with midtarsal movements painful and restricted. She was tender on pressure under the balls of the feet.

Hb 9.0 g/dl, WBC 5 X 10⁹/dl, RBC 4.0 X 10¹²/dl, ESR 44 mms/hour, serum uric acid 4.8 mg/dl, serum albumin 2.8, globulin 4.6 g/dl.

She was treated with furazolidone as above. On the fourth day the joints of the upper limbs were stiff and painful. There was pain in the neck and head. The left hip was painful and movement restricted. The left knee became swollen and stiff, but not hot. These symptoms persisted for six weeks and then suddenly disappeared and on examination six weeks later the only abnormal physical sign to be made out was some slight fluid in the supra patellar bursa above the right knee, otherwise she was without evidence of rheumatoid disease.

She was given prednisolone (enteric coated) 2.5 mgms twice daily for a week when the signs of bursitis had completely disappeared. A blood count now showed Hb 14 g/dl, WBC 6 X 10⁹/dl, RBC 4.8 X 10¹²/dl, ESR 19 mms/hour, serum albumin 5.0, globulin 3.2 g/dl. She has been on a journey to Australia and New Zealand and back lasting six months without any recurrence of symptoms and remains well.

Case 3: Female, aged 68 years. Past history: cholecystectomy for cholecystitis without gall stones. Ten years history of pains in the neck and shoulders with moderately restricted movements of the neck and shoulder joints. The neck pain tended to be severe on waking and occurred especially on the left side. Later it extended down the medial border of both scapulae, along the course of the suprascapular nerves. The joints of both middle fingers became hot, swollen, painful and the movements restricted, especially of the middle interphalangeal joints.

Examination showed moderate restriction of all movements of the neck with pain at extremes, tenderness on pressure over the cervical spine. There was audible crepitus on the neck movements and tenderness on pressure over the shoulder joints with some slight restriction and pain on movements in all directions. The interphalangeal and metacarpal-phalangeal joints of both middle fingers were hot swollen and flexion restricted, so that the tips could not voluntarily reach the palms which showed palmar erythema. X-rays of the fingers and shoulder joints were normal, but those of the neck showed mild narrowing of the disc space between C4 and C5 vertebrae.

The blood count showed an Hb 14.2g /dl, RBC 4.8 X 10¹²/dl, WBC 6 X 10⁹/dl, differential count normal, ESR 25 mms/hour, serum uric acid 4.8 mg/dl, RF (latex) positive 1 in 160, serum albumin 2.6, globulin 8.4 g/dl.

She was given furazolidone in the above dose with no effect for 4 days when she began to develop influenza-like symptoms with general malaise and aching pains in most of her joints and increased pain in the neck and shoulders and increased signs of inflammatory changes in the middle fingers, which became markedly painful and movements further restricted and the joints more swollen. She sweated slightly and ran a temperature of 39°C for 4 days. The urine became dark yellow in color. The exaggeration of symptoms of rheumatoid disease persisted for two days after cessation of treatment, at the end of which the ESR had risen to 40 mms/hour. There was no lymphadenopathy or eosinophilia. The exaggeration of symptoms then rapidly died down and within a week all symptoms and signs of rheumatoid disease had disappeared and remained absent over the next six months of observation, at the end of which time the ESR had fallen to 10 mms/hour, serum albumin 4.2, globulin 2.8 g/dl. She now feels extremely well.

Case 4: Female, aged 43 years. Her mother suffers from rheumatoid arthritis and diabetes. Past history: nil revelant.

Rheumatoid disease began some 5 months before being seen with pain in the balls of the feet on weight bearing, the feet swelling and the midtarsal joints becoming painful. The toes were painful on flexion and the ankles painful on any movement. Two years previously she had pains across the lower abdomen and lumbar spine, which have persisted. In the last three months pains and swelling had spread to the fingers, thumbs, wrists, shoulders and neck, which was stiff. She suffered from night sweats. There was marked morning stiffness. RF was positive. She had been treated elsewhere with aspirin, Indocid® and exercise with some relief.

Examination showed warmth, tenderness, swelling and restricted movements of the wrists, finger joints, thumb joints and both midtarsal joints with tenderness on pressure under the metatarsals. X-rays showed no bony changes.

She was treated with metronidazole 2 Gm on two successive evenings which was followed by generalized joint pains after 24 hours with sweating, headache, and a temperature of 38.6°C. Seven weeks later there was marked improvement in her symptoms, but the thumb and first finger joint on both sides remained hot and swollen and the tips could not be flexed into the palms. Otherwise there were no abnormal physical signs. ESR was 45 mms/hour, Hb 10 g/dl, serum albumin 2.6, globulin 8.2 g/dl, serum uric acid 4.8 mg/dl.

The symptoms persisted over the next two months when the dose of metronidazole was repeated with a similar result. After a further two months her only symptoms were pains on the dorsum of the fingers and tenderness of the right sternoclavicular joint. Five months later she noticed some return of pains and swelling to the fingers and wrists and hotness and tenderness of the right sternoclavicular joint, and hotness and tenderness on the inner side of the left foot, which could not be inverted fully without pain. The symptoms remained unchanged requiring treatment with aspirin for the next year. At this time the ESR was 25 mms/hour.

She was treated with furazolidone as above. After three days this caused aching in the fingers, elbows and shoulders and the midtarsal joints with generalized influenza-like symptoms and tenderness in most of the other joints. She sweated and her temperature rose to 38.2°C for 3 days. The ESR rose to 80 mms/hour. Her symptoms rapidly disappeared three days after cessation of treatment when she complained of only occasional sharp pains in various joints, but there were no physical signs of rheumatoid disease to be made out. Four months after being treated with furazolidone the ESR had fallen to 12 mms/hour, blood count showed Hb 15 g/dl. Over the course of the next three months she became completely symptomless and has remained so for eight months since the course of furazolidone, with serum albumin 4.0, globulin 3.0 g/dl.

Case 5: Male, aged 53 years. Grandmother and mother both suffered from rheumatoid arthritis. Nil significant in the past history.

For 15 years he had suffered from pain in the back of the right wrist with swelling, hotness and difficulty in dorsiflexion. There was occasional similar pain in the left wrist. RF was positive. A blood count and ESR were completely normal and serum uric acid was 4.2 mg/dl. X-rays of the wrists and hands showed no bony changes. He was treated with Indocid® 25 mg twice daily which controlled the swelling, but did not completely relieve the pain and had no affect on the restriction of wrist movement. He had also been treated by acupuncture and some kind of electrical stimulation of the area without benefit and various herbal remedies without effect. A notable feature was that the pain and swelling were worse in the morning after taking alcohol of any sort.

On examination of the dorsum of the right wrist and neighbouring region of the hand was markedly swollen, hot and tender in one small area. No dorsiflexion of the wrist was possible and palmar flexion and lateral deviation of the wrists was somewhat limited. No rheumatoid changes were found elsewhere in the body.

He was treated with furazolidone as above and this was followed by a marked increase in the swelling in the dorsum of the right wrist lasting 14 days. He also had slight symptoms affecting the left wrist. Three weeks after taking the tablets pain and swelling had ceased and the movements of the wrists had returned to normal for the first time in 15 years. He has been followed for six months without return of symptoms or signs. The ESR and RF have not yet been retested.

Case 6: Male, aged 59 years. Family and past history nil revelant.

Two months before being seen he noticed an onset of marked weakness of the arms with stiffness of the wrists and fingers, which could not be extended fully, and an inability to make a fist on either side. He also had tingling in the inner side of the thumb, index and middle fingers and the outer side of the ring finger on both hands. The neck was somewhat stiff and there was marked pain and restricted movements of both shoulders and in the elbows, especially the left, and these could not be extended fully. There was also some pain and restricted flexion of the right knee. There was marked sweating of the palms of the hands, especially on the right. All the symptoms were worse after sitting. X-rays at another hospital showed no abnormalities in the joints. The weakness of the upper limbs were so severe that he was unable to carry on his work as a pianist. RF in the serum was mildly positive.

A blood count showed Hb 13.0 gm/dl, WBC 6 X 10^4/dl, RBC 3.8 X 10^6/dl, ESR 44 mms/hour, serum uric acid 5.8 mg/dl, serum albumin 3.0, globulin 4.8 g/dl. He had been treated at another hospital for four months with indomethacin 25 mg three times daily without benefit.

Examination showed marked weakness of all muscles of the arms and of movements of the wrists and fingers with inability to lift his arms above an angle of 75° of the body at the shoulders. He was unable to dress or undress because of this weakness. The palms were sweating profusely and on both sides there was evidence of median nerve dysfunction. The finger joints and wrists were swollen, hot and markedly restricted. He was unable to flex the index and ring fingers into the palms. Both elbow joints were hot and tender and the movements restricted and there was marked tenderness and pain on attempted movement of the shoulder joints. Movements were partly restricted by severe weakness and pain. There were no abnormalities in the lower limbs. The CNS was normal, but a tensilon test was positive indicating the presence of myasthenia gravis in addition to bilateral median nerve dysfunction evidently associated with the rheumatoid condition.

He was treated with furazolidone as above. This produced a headache on the second day when all his joints became painful and there was general malaise, aching and morning stiffness. He sweated during sleep, but nine days after commencing treatment there was a rapid improvement in the joint pains and weakness of his upper limbs, though three weeks later he was still unable to close his fingers fully and full extension of the right wrist was not completely possible. There was also slight weakness of extension of the right elbow.

Two months after treatment he still complained of stiffness on waking and after sitting with occasional pain in the right shoulder, both elbows and the middle interphalangeal joint of the right index finger. He was not quite able to make a fist and the medial nerve disturbances were still present. The middle interphalangeal joints of both index fingers were slightly swollen and tender with restricted flexion. The course of furazolidone was then repeated for 7 days again with mild increase in pains in the upper limb joints with hotness and swelling of the wrists and elbows and increased pain in the right shoulder joint lasting for 5 days, after which the myasthenic symptoms had completely disappeared and the symptoms of medial nerve dysfunction were absent. All joint pain and swelling had now ceased. He has been followed for a further six months and has remained symptomless. The ESR now had fallen to 9 mms/hour, serum Hb 15 gm/dl, WBC 5 X 10⁹/dl, RBC 5.5 X 10¹²/dl, serum albumin 6.8, globulin 2.8 gm/dl.

Successive cases treated with allopurinol

Case 1: Male, aged 66 years. Fifteen year history of pain, swelling and restricted movements, particularly of knees, but also of hips, ankles, wrists and hands. He had been treated by many anti-inflammatory drugs including aspirin, Naprosyn®, indomethacin, Motril®, brufen and others. None of these helped the pain and swelling of the joints.

On examination there was heat, swelling and restricted movements, especially affecting the knees but also the ankles, midtarsal joints, elbows, wrists, both shoulder joints and the neck. The finger joints were swollen, hot and tender and he could not make a fist on either side. RF in the serum was strongly positive, the ESR was 40 mms/hour, Hb 11 gm/dl, RBC 4.0 X 10¹²/dl, WBC 6 X 10⁹/dl, serum uric acid 5.6 mg/dl, serum albumin 3.0, globulin 4.2 gm/dl. Differential count was normal.

He was treated with allopurinol 300 mg, three times daily for 7 days without any reaction until the 4th day when he began to get shooting pains in most of his joints. The temperature rose to 39.2-39.4° C for 5 days accompanied by shivering chills and on the 6th day by profuse sweating, severe stabbing pains affected the whole lower limbs, but also in various other parts of the body. This lasted for 9 days when his temperature settled and remained normal.

Five weeks after the initial rise in temperature his symptoms and signs of disease had completely disappeared according to him "in a most extraordinary way."

He has been followed for eight months during which time he has had no return of rheumatoid symptoms. He is playing golf, tennis, squash racquets and swimming. His ESR is now 5 mm/hour, HB 15.2/dl, RBC 5.3 X 10¹²/dl, WBC 6.5 X 10⁹/dl, RF negative, serum uric acid 4.6 mg/dl, serum albumin 6.2, globulin 3.2 gm/dl.

Case 2: Male, aged 22 years. Family history — Grandfather suffered from rheumatoid arthritis. Three years previously the patient's right knee became painful and swollen and the left knee, both ankles and left elbow followed within the next six weeks. These symptoms were relieved by brufen and paracetemol during the next six months, but after two years he developed pain in the lumbar region and pain, swelling, hotness and restricted movements of the right elbow and wrist and then other joints became affected on the left. Iridocyclitis appeared. This had varied in severity over the next year during which time the left shoulder and neck became painful with restricted movments and then the hips and the heels and insteps were also painful. He sweated excessively and the back of the neck was stiff. He had been treated with seven (7) 25 mg tablets of Indocid® and 6 paracetemol a day. The London Hospital had informed him that he had ankylosing spondylitis.

Examination showed some slight painful restriction movements to right and left. All movements of the left shoulder were moderately restricted by pain. Extension of the right elbow was limited to 15° with pain. The right wrist was hot, swollen and all movements restricted. Other joints were not affected. There was no evidence of iritis at the time.

He was treated with metronidazole 2 Gm on two successive evenings which resulted in influenza-like symptoms on the first two days and on the second day exaggeration of the pain and swelling by pain in both shoulder joints, right toes, balls of the feet and heels on weight bearing. After this the elbows were less painful and their movements less restricted. Other joints however were not infected. He had continued to take Indocid® and paracetemol during this time.

One month after taking metronidazole there was slight pain at the back of the neck on flexion, but movements were full. The shoulder joints were normal. The elbows were painless and would now straighten almost completely. The right wrist was cold and not tender and the movements were now full.

The treatment was repeated and six weeks later the only symptom was slight pain in the ball of the right foot when walking.

He remained well during the next two years without taking any anti-inflammatory drugs when he reported that for the last two weeks his left shoulder had begun to ache and both knees gave him some pain on walking. The right elbow became painful and could not be extended fully. His neck was stiff on waking. There was generalized morning stiffness.

Examination showed the right elbow could not be fully extended by 10°. The blood count was normal, but the ESR was 30 mms/hour. RF was negative, serum uric acid was 5.2 mg/dl, serum albumin 4.1, globulin 5.2 gm/dl.

He was treated with allopurinol 300 mg three times daily for 7 days. This produced mild influenza-like symptoms, slight pyrexia of 38.2°C and some generalized joint pains especially for the right elbow and left shoulder joints and swelling of both wrists lasting for two days.

Following this the symptoms rapidly disappeared and within two weeks of beginning treatment he was completely symptomless without any physical signs of disease. The ESR had fallen to 9 mms/hour one month after beginning treatment with allopurinol.

He has remained completely well over the last nine months. Serum albumin 5.0, gloublin 2.8 gm/dl now.

Case 3: Female, aged 64 years. White inhabitant of Barbados. Family history, mother suffered from cholecystitis and mild rheumatoid arthritis and half-sister from thryotoxicosis and a sister died of gastro-intestinal cancer.

In 1967 she had several attacks of cystitis and in June 1969 mild pains and swelling of the finger joints, wrists and pains and restricted movements of the shoulders and ankles. She was treated with aspirin without benefit and in 1970 she began to suffer from severe weakness and arthropathy of almost all the joints and an anaemia requiring blood transfusions. She was treated by repeated courses of gold injections until 1972 when this was changed to prednisolone and indomethacin suppositories. In 1974 she had a replacement of the right hip carried out. In 1974 both knees had become severely affected with the disease. In 1978 she began to suffer from recurrent chest infections and perennial "hay-fever". In 1978 the pain and restricted movements of the neck became so severe that an x-ray was taken and showed severe involvement of the whole cervical spine with subluxation of C1 on C2 vertebra, for which she was treated with a collar. The movements of the shoulders became remarkably painful and restricted with nodules round the elbows. In 1979 there was severe pain under the balls of the feet and she developed nasal blocking at this time. There was a slight chest cough with brown sputum. There was pain in the right chest on deep breathing. She also complained of considerable generalized pruritus.

Examination in 1979 showed bilateral nasal congestion, severe thinness, the chest exhibited crepitations in the right mid-zone, movements of the neck were impossible and the elbows and wrists were severely painful with all movements restricted with nodules round the elbow. The fingers and thumbs were completely useless with ankylosed joints. The right hip movements were free and painless (the site of the prosthesis) and the left hip movements were markedly painful and restricted. The knees were knobbly without free fluid, but with severe crepitus and full movements accompanied by pain. The midtarsal joints were fixed. The toes were markedly involved with over-riding. She was unable to stand. X-rays of the chest showed diffuse shadowing in the right lung. The serum Hb was 10 gm/dl, RBC 11 X 10⁶/dl, WBC 7.0 X 10⁴/dl, differential count normal, serum uric acid 5.5 mg/dl, ESR 88 mms/hr, serum albumin 1.8, globulin 5.8 gm/dl. X-rays showed gross destruction of the knees, left hip joint, fingers, wrists and elbows and of the midtarsal joints with gross deformities of the toes. The RF was strongly positive. An ophthalmological opinion showed a positive Shirmer's test on both sides with evidence of scleritis and conjunctivitis.

She was treated with allopurinol as above and at the same time clobetasone butyrate 0.1% drops for the eyes 2-4 times daily.

In four days she began to run an evening pyrexia of 39.2-39.4°C and complained of pain, hotness and swelling of most joints and pain in the neck. In addition she developed rheumatoid nodules over the sacrum and on the dorsa of both feet. The increase in symptoms lasted for two weeks when the pyrexia settled and the rheumatoid nodules began to disappear slowly. The pain in the neck gradually lessened and the hotness of the joints died down. By this time the movements of the neck showed marked improvement in all directions and those of the shoulders improved to such an extent she was able to do her hair and feed herself again. She was able to walk round the room, but this produced aching in the knee joints after five minutes. There was, however, no joint swelling and her temperature had fallen to normal.

This improvement was maintained over the next eight months and at the end of this time the serum Hb was 13.8 gm/dl, the ESR had fallen to 19 mms/hour, RBC was 4.6 X 10⁶/dl, serum uric acid 4.6 mm/dl, serum albumin 5.8, globulin 3.6 gm/dl. The eyes were markedly less dry as confirmed by Shirmer's test and there was no evidence of active rheumatoid disease, though the previous articular damage, of course, persisted.

Case 4: Female, aged 63 years. Family history nil revelant. Past history hysterectomy for fibroids and bilateral ovarian cystestomy aged 49 years. Ten years later she fell and injured the right ankle and immediately developed pain, hotness, swelling and restricted movements of the fingers, thumbs, wrists, knees, elbows, shoulders, hips and ankles, pain and stiffness and restricted movements of the neck and pain under the balls of the feet when weight bearing. This was accompanied by occipital headaches, sweating and loss of weight.

In addition she later developed symptoms of ulcerative colitis proven by sigmoidoscopy, radiological appearances and mucosal biopsy. She was treated by numerous anti-inflammatory substances, including indomethacin, Naprosyn®, Felden®, Froben®, brufen, gold injections and then by penicillamine and prednisolone and later by prednisolone and salazopyrin for the colitis. None of these produced appreciable improvement in her condition.

Her blood showed Hb 10.0 gm/dl, WBC 7500 X 10⁴/dl, ESR 55 mms/hour, RF strongly positive, serum uric acid 5.3 mg/dl, albumin 4.2 gm/dl, globulin 6.3 gm/dl.

Examination showed high facial color with mild mucosal pallor, mild rheumatoid deformities of wrists and fingers, left olecranon bursitis, pain and restricted movements of the shoulders, elbows, wrists, neck, marked crepitus during movements of both knee joints with restricted flexion and the presence of free fluid. Movements were painful at the extremes. The left ankle showed pain on extension and she was tender on pressure under the balls of the feet. Walking was painful at the knees and under the balls of the feet. She was tender over the large intestine.

She was treated with allopurinol as above. After 4 days this produced an increase in the symptoms of arthropathy with pain in the hips, knees and ankles, the two latter becoming hot and swollen and her neck painful on movment. Her temperature rose on the 4th day to 38.5°C and there was general malaise and influenza-like symptoms. The muscles were tender to the touch and she sweated profusely.

These symptoms continued until two days after cessation of the drug administration when the temperature suddenly fell to normal and within 5 days there was a complete cessation of all joint swelling, hotness and pain and cessation of symptoms and signs of ulcerative colitis.

One month later the serum Hb had risen to 13.8 gm/dl, ESR had fallen to 22 mms/hour, serum uric acid 5.4 mg/dl.

The temperature remained completely normal and she has remained symptomless without taking any drugs over the last ten months and without any visual evidence of arthritis, bursitis or deformities. No intestinal symptoms and barium enema normal. Serum albumin 6.4 gm/dl, globulin 4.0 gm/dl.

Case 5: Female, aged 60 years. Family history — no rheumatoid disease. Eighteen months previously she began to notice pain, swelling, hotness and restricted movements of the fingers and wrists later spreading to the elbows, shoulders and neck and to the knees, ankles and midtarsal joints with pain under the balls of the feet on weight bearing. She had been previously treated with indomethacin and aspirin without relief. On examination there was evidence of acute active inflammation in the fingers, thumbs, wrists, elbows and shoulder joints with pain, tenderness, heat and restricted movements. The neck movements were painful and restricted. She was unable to extend her elbows fully or to do up or undo her brassiere. She could not feed herself. The wrists, fingers and thumb joints were markedly swollen, hot and tender and she was unable to make a fist on either side. The knees were hot, swollen with free fluid and restricted flexion and this also applied to the ankles and metatarsal joints.

Hb was 10.2 gm/dl, WBC 8 X 10^9/dl, RBC 4.0 X 10^{12}/dl, ESR 42 mms/hour, serum uric acid 4.4 mg/dl, serum albumin 4.9 gm/dl, globulin 6.2 gm/dl, RF positive.

She was treated with allopurinol as above which produced on the third day a marked rise in temperature to 39.5° C, sweating and generalized pains in the muscles and joints which became swollen and hot and included the temporo-mandibular joints. The symptoms were severe enough to interfere with sleep in spite of continuing with the Naprosyn® as before treatment.

Ten days after beginning treatment there was a sudden fall in temperature and evidence of active rheumatoid arthritis rapidly disappeared, so that after ten days she was completely free of pain, stiffness on waking and one month after beginning treatment she showed no abnormal physical signs whatsoever.

After three months repetition of blood tests showed Hb 14.6 gm/dl, RC 4.8 X10^{12}, ESR 16 mms/hour, serum uric acid 5.6 mg/dl, serum albumin 6.4 gm/dl, globulin 5.6 gm/dl.

She has been followed for a further six months without return of symptoms or recourse to pain killing drugs.

Case 6: Female, aged 54 years, Brazilian. Family history — mother suffered from rheumatoid arthritis. Eight years previous to being seen she began to complain of pain, hotness, swelling and restricted movements of the fingers, wrists, elbows and shoulders, both knees, especially the right, left ankle and midtarsal joints. This had been treated in Brazil by hot wax baths to the fingers and wrists, by massage, exercising of the upper limbs, hands and lower limbs and by various anti-inflammatory drugs, including prednisolone 5 mgms twice daily, none of which have controlled the symptoms.

On examination there were typical rheumatoid arthritic changes in the above mentioned joints with swelling and heat, marked palmar erythema with restricted extension of the right knee. There was tenderness on pressure under the balls of the feet and bilateral olecranon bursitis. Neck movements were restricted with tenderness on pressure over the cervical spine at the side of the neck. She was unable to raise her arms above the shoulder, walking was only possible with a stick.

X-rays showed a minimal loss of disc space between C5-6 vertebrae in the neck, but were otherwise normal. Blood showed strongly positive RF, ESR 104 mms/hour, Hb 10 gm/dl, WBC 5 X 10⁹/dl, RBC 4 X 10¹²/dl, serum uric acid 4.6 mg/dl, serum albumin 2.0 gm/dl, globulin 5.8 gm/dl. The temperature was 38.0°C and there was palmar erythema and sweating.

Treatment consisted of gradually tapering off the prednisolone and substituting with Felden® 2 tablets in the morning. This, however, did not control the symptoms. She was therefore treated with a course of allopurinol.

Within three days she had a violent joint reaction with pain, swelling, hotness and restricted movements of all her joints, profuse sweating and considerable pain requiring morphine injections to control it. The temperature reached 40.0°C for several days.

After ten days there was a sudden cessation of her joint symptoms, pain and sweating and a fall in the temperature.

Within a week she was free of any joint symptoms and was able to walk normally. At the height of her symptoms the ESR had risen to 140 mms/hour, WBC 9 X 10⁹/dl and 8% eosinophilia.

She was observed for the next six months during which time the symptoms did not return, even after giving up anti-inflammatory drugs.

The serum uric acid was at that time 4.6 mg/dl, Hb 14.5 gm/dl and the ESR was 18 mms/hour, serum albumin 6.8 gm/dl, globulin 5 gm/dl.

Conclusion

The above findings show that when the antiamoebic substances *furazolidone* and *allopurinol* are administered to patients suffering from active rheumatoid disease, within a few days they cause an exaggeration of the disease symptoms, which may be severe and accompanied by a rise in ESR, eosinophilia, sweating, pyrexia, all of which begin to die down after about ten days. This may be sudden and is followed by rapid and complete relief of disease symptoms providing there has not been destruction of joint cartilage or bone or deformities have been present. Myasthenia gravis and ulcerative colitis likewise disappear.

In the next six months all serological signs of infection disappear and the patient returns to health with normalization of the ESR and the Hb and in the course of time the RF becomes negative. The exaggeration of symptoms is an example of the Jarisch-Herxheimer reaction. This is in accord with the previous demonstration of the presence of a free-living amoeba in the region of the joints and elsewhere in the body and of the curative effect of other antiamoebic substances, such as 5-nitronimidazoles.

(Based on Madden, J.E., B.M., B. Ch. [Oxford],
and
Mendel D., M.D., B.S.
Hounslow Health Centre, Middlesex, England)
The effect of tinidazole on cases of active
rheumatoid arthritis[2],[3],[4].

Introduction

Wyburn-Mason (1978) first reported the effect of 5-nitroimidazole drugs on cases of active rheumatoid arthritis. He found that in almost all cases, on first administration, they caused an immediate transient exaggeration of the manifestations of the disease often with influenza-like symptoms and in the appearance of lesions in tissues not previously affected. These symptoms gradually disappeared over the course of the next 2-3 months and in many cases all signs of disease activity were lost both clinically and serologically in the course of 8-12 months. The exaggeration of the symptoms of the disease could be lessened by the concomittant administration of an anti-inflammatory substance.

The authors undertook a trial in an attempt to confirm this report, using the most potent antiprotozoal drug of the 5-nitroimidazole series, namely tinidazole. The cases of rheumatoid arthritis used in the trial were successive ones fulfilling the features of probable, definite or classical examples according to the American Rheumatism Association classification encountered in a general medical practice. In most cases those which were already taking anti-inflammatory drugs continued on this regime and the tinidazole was given as 2 gram doses on 2 successive days. An attempt at a double blind crossover trial with a placebo was unsuccessful, since in all cases taking tinidazole within 24 hours there occurred generalized malaise with influenza-like symptoms, profuse nocturnal sweating and a marked increase in the arthropathy by the second or third day so that the trial was no longer blind to the observer. Instead of this an open trial was used. Full investigations of each case were carried out immediately before and throughout the trial and continued for 12 months or more after the administration of the tinidazole. All patients were advised not to take alcohol during the next month and not to exercise the joints any more than was essential and to avoid massage and heating the joints.

Successive cases treated with tinidazole

Case 1: Female, aged 54 years. Family history nil revelant. Acute onset of painful joint swelling in October 1979 involving the fingers, wrists, shoulders, knees and feet. Treated with aspirin without improvement.

Examination showed painful, tender, hot swelling of the wrists, finger and thumb joints, knees and ankles. Serum ANF positive, RF negative, ESR 20 mms per hour. HB 14.6 Gm per cent. RBC 4.4 ml X 10^{12}/dl, WBC 5.8 X 10^9/dl, no LE cells, albumin 2.4 mm per cent, globulin 2.4 mms per cent. Radiographs of wrists, fingers, knees, ankles normal.

On January 15th and 16th 1980 she was treated with 2 grams of tinidazole on both days. This resulted in influenza-like symptoms lasting 36 hours with severe nocturnal sweats and some increase in the severity of the arthropathy lasting for 10 days following which there was a rapid disappearance of the joint swelling, pain and heat and return of the movements to normal during the next 12 months.

After six months she was completely symptomless. The ESR was 14 mm per hour. ANF and RF were still positive. Hb was 14.8 Gm/dl, RBC 4.8 x 10^{12}/dl, WBC 5.5 X 10^9/dl, serum albumin 3.0 Gm per cent, globulin 1.8 Gm per cent. Eighteen months after treatment apart from occasional joint pains varying with the climate and controlled by aspirin she has remained well. The ESR is now 6 mm/hour, ANF and RF negative.

Case 2: Male, aged 43 years. Family history nil revelant. Twelve year history of progressive seropositive rheumatoid arthritis beginning in the wrists and gradually spreading to involve the fingers, ankles, knees, elbows, shoulders, neck and midtarsal joints. He had been treated with indomethacin and prednisolone throughout.

Examination showed typical rheumatoid changes in all the above joints with signs of activity as evidenced by heat and pain. All the joint movements were restricted, especially wrists, fingers and knees, which exhibited free fluid in the joint cavities. The arms could not be raised about 45° at the shoulders and he was unable to shave, feed himself, do up his tie or put on his coat. Walking was painful and limited and movements of the knees and ankles were restricted and of the midtarsal joints non-existent. He could not make a fist and dorsiflexion and palmar flexion of the wrists was impossible. The fingers and thumbs could not be fully extended. X-rays showed loss of joint space in both knees and fingers. Serum ANF negative, latex test positive 1 in 20, RAHA positive 1 in 2560, ESR 64 mm per hour, Hb 11.0 Gm per cent, RBC 4.2 X 10^{12}/l, WBC 10.9 X 10^9/l, neutrophils 59 per cent, lymphocytes 33 per cent, albumin 1.8 Gm per cent, globulin 3.8 Gm per cent, IgG 2000 mg/dl, IgA 500 mg/dl, IgM 200 mg/dl.

On 2nd and 3rd of February 1980 he was treated with tinidazole 2 grams on both days. He continued on indomethacin and prednisolone. This resulted in some exaggeration of his symptoms over the first week followed by a definite lessening of the pain and hotness of the joints and after two months the ESR had fallen to 19 mms per hour, RAHA was positive 1 in 640, latex test positive 1 in 20 and the ANF was negative.

Because of the improvement the patient requested another course of treatment three months after the first. This was given as 2 grams tinidazole on the 1st and 2nd April 1980 and was followed by headache, general malaise and an increase in the joint pains a week later. He was tapered off steroids.

Six months later there was a remarkable improvement and all signs of activity of the disease were absent, the joints being cold and mostly painless, not swollen and with full movements, except for the knees which were still painful with marked crepitus on movements due to secondary osteoarthritic changes, and some pain and swelling of the finger joints.

One year after the first treatment with tinidazole the ANF was negative, the RF latex test was less than 1 in 20 and the RAHA was now 1 in 80, albumin as 3.6 Gm per cent, globulin 2.8 Gm per cent, ESR was 19 mms per hour, Hb 14.8 g per cent. RBC 4.6 X $10^{12}/1$, WBC 7.8 X $10^9/1$. He has remained symptomless apart from his knees and fingers and is still under observation.

Case 3: Female, aged 50 years. Family history, nil revelant. Three year history of gradual increase in pain, swelling, hotness and restricted movements of fingers, wrists, elbows, shoulders, neck, temporo-mandibular joints, knees, ankles, midtarsal joints and metatarso-phalangeal joints in spite of treatment with aspirin, gold injections, levamisole, indomethacin and opren.

On examination there was typical rheumatoid arthritis affecting the fingers and thumb joints, wrists, elbows, shoulders, knee joints with effusions, ankles and midtarsal joints with oedema of the feet and inability to move either the ankles or midtarsal joints. Joint x-rays showed no cartilage or bony damage. Serum ANF negative, RF latex positive 1 in 640, Rose Waaler test positive 1 in 64, ESR 34 mms per hour, serum albumin 2.8 Gm per 100 ml, globulin 3.8 g per 100 ml, IgG 2000 mg/dl, IgA 400 mg/dl, IgM 200 mg/dl, Hb 12.0 Gm/d, RBC 3.5 X $10^{12}/1$.

She continued to take opren, but on January 9 and 10, 1980, she took 2 Gm tinidazole each evening. This was followed by influenza-like symptoms and general exaggeration of arthropathy over the next three weeks followed by gradual general improvement.

After two months evidence of active joint disease had disappeared and she began to put on weight and the muscle power to improve. After six months the ESR was 18 mms per hour.

She had given up treatment with opren and after one year was completely symptomless except for occasional joint pain after twisting or wrenching or with changes in the weather. At this time serum albumin was 4.0 Gm per cent, globulin 2.5 Gm per cent, IgG 800 mg/dl, IgA 60 mg/dl, IgM 140 mg/dl, ESR 6 mms/hour.

She has remained symptomless while still being followed two years after initial treatment.

Case 4: Female aged 73 years. Family history a sister suffered from severe rheumatoid arthritis. The patient gave a ten year history of progressive pain, swelling, hotness of fingers, wrists, elbows, shoulders, neck, knees, ankles and midtarsal joints with considerable pain on the balls of the feet when weight bearing. There was pain in the region of the temporo-mandibular joints when chewing. She had been taking brufen over the last year with no appreciable relief of symptoms.

Examination showed tenderness on pressure over the temporo-mandibular joints, restricted painful movements of the head on the neck in all directions with pain on pressure over the cervical spine, marked restriction and pain of the shoulder movements bilaterally with tenderness on pressure over joint spaces. The elbows were swollen, hot and tender and could not be fully extended or flexed. Both wrists were swollen, very tender with marked restriction of all movements with swelling of the meta-carpophalangeal and interphalangeal joints of all fingers. She was unable to make a fist or to extend the fingers fully. Palmar erythema was present; marked weakness of all movements of the upper limbs. The knee joints were swollen, hot and tender at the joint spaces with crepitus more marked on the left. Both ankle joints showed with bony thickening and restricted movements, midtarsal joints were swollen, hot and tender with absent movements. There was tenderness on pressure under the heads of all the metatarsals, some general oedema of the feet and ankles. Blood examination — ANF, RF strongly positive. ESR 62 mms/hr, Hb 11.4 Gm/dl, RBC 4.3 X $10^{12}/1$, WBC 30 X $10^9/1$, 67 per cent neutrophils, 25 per cent lymphocytes, 4 per cent monocytes, 4 per cent eosinophils, albumin 2.1 Gm per cent, globulin 4.3 Gm per cent. X-rays showed losses of joint spaces in the knees and interphalangeal joints of the fingers. IgG 3000 mg/dl, IgA 550 mg/dl, IgM 200 mg/dl.

On January 11th and 12th 1980 she was given tinidazole 2 grams on two successive evenings. Brufen was continued, but the tinidazole produced an influenza-like reaction with sweating and pyrexia of 38.8°C on the next two days and some exaggeration of joint pain and swelling.

She was seen again on May 20th 1980 when there was a remarkable improvement in her general condition. The hotness and swelling of all the joints had disappeared. The neck and jaw ache were no longer present. The shoulder, neck and elbow movements were full and painless. The wrist swelling had disappeared. The joints were no longer hot and movements were almost normal, the finger movements were no longer painful and swelling almost disappeared. Flexion and extension of metacarphophalangeal and interphalangeal joints were full with normal grip. The hip joints were normal. The knee joints were no longer swollen or hot, but movements were still painful. The swelling of the feet was no longer present and movements of the ankles and midtarsal joints were full, free and painless. There was still tenderness on pressure over the heads of the metatarsals.

On May 7th 1980 the blood showed ANF and RF negative, ESR 3 mm/hr, Hb 14.6 gm/l, RBC 4.8 X 10^{12}/dl, WBC 4.1 X 10^9/l 46 per cent neutrophils, 46 per cent lymphocytes, 5 per cent monocytes, 3 per cent eosinophils, albumen 4.5 Gm per cent, globulin 2.3 Gm per cent.

On December 5th 1981 she remained symptomless apart from the secondary osteoarthritic symptoms in both knees. The serum protein showed albumen 4.6 Gm per cent, globulin 2.4 Gm per cent, IgG 1000 mg/dl, IgA 300 mg/dl, IgM 110 mg/dl. She remains under observation and symptomless except for some pains in both knees.

Case 5: Male aged 69 years. Family history — mother suffered from asthma. At the age of 35 years the patient developed nocturnal asthma. Ten years previous to being seen he developed pains in the upper arms after exercise and drenching night sweats to be followed by calf pains on exertion and eventually generalized pains in the muscles which became tender and wasted. These symptoms became much worse two years before being seen. He also noticed painful lumps under the skin lasting 24 hours, morning stiffness, pains, hotness, swelling and restricted movements of the elbows and knees and pain and stiffness of the back of the neck. The shoulders became stiff and their movements painful and greatly restricted as were the wrists, fingers and thumbs. Also, pain was present in both hip joints and pain, swelling, hotness and restricted movements of both ankles, midtarsal joints and pains under the balls of both feet. The left toes became deformed. He also suffered recurrent left painful parotid swelling. He had been treated by recurrent courses of gold injections over 8 years, indomethacin 100 mg and 8 soluble aspirin a day over many years without control of the pain and progress of the disease. He was now completely helpless.

Examination showed blood pressure 100/120, left parotid gland markedly swollen and tender. All movements of the neck grossly restricted and painful and there was marked tenderness over the cervical vertebrae. All the shoulder joint movements grossly restricted and painful. He was unable to get his hand to his mouth to feed himself, shave or comb his hair or to take his shirt or coat on or off. All elbow movements were grossly restricted by pain and tenderness of joints which were hot. The wrists were swollen, hot and all movements impossible because of pain. Finger and thumb joints were thickened, cold and movements slight and restricted. He was unable to write, cut up his food, dress himself or go to the toilet. The knees were normal. Both ankles and midtarsal joints were thickened, hot and movements were impossible. The left toes showed outward deviation with tenderness under the balls of the feet on pressure. The palms were red.

62

He was unable to walk more than a few paces. Serum RF positive 1 in 640, ESR 102 mms/hr, ANF positive, Hb 9.4 Gm per 100 ml, RBC 4.2 x 10^{12}/1, WBC 7.6 x 10^9/1, differential count normal, serum albumin 1.8 Gm per 100 ml, globulin 4.6 Gm per 100 ml, IgG 2400 mg/dl, IgA 450 mg/dl, IgM 210 mg/dl. He then developed persistent diarrhoea with the passage of mucus and blood. Sigmoidoscopy and rectal biopsy and a barium enema showed typical ulcerative colitis. The indomethacin and aspirin were continued.

On April 6th and 7th 1980 he was given tinidazole 2 Gm on each occasion. This resulted in a violent reaction with further swelling and pain in the left parotid gland and pyrexia of 39°C, drenching night sweats, headache, severe neck pain and stiffness and a generalized increase in pain, swelling and stiffness in all the joints in the body. The shoulders were so markedly affected he was unable to move his arms at the shoulders as though paralysed. Within a week the pyrexia and sweating had ceased and the pain, swelling and hotness of the joints began to decrease.

After four weeks there was considerable improvement in all his symptoms and at that time the ESR was 140 mm per hour. The parotid swelling had disappeared.

Over the next twelve months there was a gradual disappearance of all signs of active disease. His diarrhoea and abdominal pain ceased. Power returned to his limbs and the muscle wasting lessened until he was left with only some bony thickening of the left ankle. He was now able to look after himself in the normal fashion, eat, feed, shave and dress himself and to walk normally. He began to gain weight and the ESR now was 19 mms per hour. The blood pressure had fallen to 140/80. He had been able to give up taking aspirin, indomethacin and some five months previously the ANF and RF were negative, Hb 15.2 Gm/dl, RBC 4.8 X 10^{12}/1, WBC 6.8 X 10^9/1, differential count normal, albumin 3.2 Gm per cent, globulin 2.8 Gm per cent, IgG 1200 mg/dl, IgA 280 mg/dl, IgM 80 mg/dl, barium enema was normal.

He has remained symptomless and under continued observation without further treatment during 2 years.

Case 6: Female, aged 45 years. Six months history of progressive pain, hotness, swelling and restricted movements of wrists and knees, night sweats, morning stiffness and occipital headaches.

Examination showed palmar erythema, swelling, tenderness, heat and restricted movements of wrists and knees with free fluid in the latter. Blood count showed Hb 12.6 Gm per cent, ESR 42 mms per hour, RF positive 1 in 320, serum albumin 1.8 Gm/dl, IgG 2000 mg/dl, IgA 350 mg/dl, IgM 200 mg/dl, LE cells negative, Rose Waaler 1 in 32. She was treated with brufen tablets 2 three times daily after meals during six months with some lessening of the pain and heat, but no obvious regression of arthropathy. Fluid persisted in the knee joints.

On January 8th 1980 she was treated with tinidazole 2 Gm on 2 successive evenings. After three hours she noticed influenza-like symptoms with exaggeration of the heat, pain and swelling of the wrists and knees and the appearance of similar symptoms in the fingers and ankles. There was marked sweating during sleep. Brufen was continued.

The exaggeration of symptoms was maximal on the third day after tinidazole was given and thereafter gradual improvment over the next two months when the arthropathy had disappeared and the patient felt well. The ESR was now 68 mms per hour. Six months later she still remained symptomless in spite of giving up brufen and the ESR had fallen to 9 mms per hour, the RF was now negative and the blood Hb had risen to 14.8 Gm dl. A year after treatment the serum IgG was 1400 mg/dl, IgA 330 mg/dl, IgM 100 mg/dl.

She is still under observation and symptomless and requires no treatment.

Case 7: Male, aged 49 years. Onset of swelling, pain and restricted movements of the left metacarpo-carpal joint of the thumb persisting for six months followed by acute onset of intense pain and restricted movements of the left shoulder joint making it impossible for him to dress himself. This persisted for five months and was followed by pain in the right shoulder and in the right metacarpo-carpal joint of the thumb.

Examination showed signs of gross pain on attempted movement of both shoulder joints which could not be raised forward or laterally more than 45°. The metacarpo-carpal joints of the thumbs were severly tender and movements impossible. X-rays of the shoulder joints and thumbs were normal. ESR 36 mms/hr, RF positive, albumin 2 Gm/dl, globulin 2 Gm/dl. He was treated with 2 Gm tinidazole on two successive evenings with violent sweating on each night and increased pain in the affected joints making it impossible for him to look after himself.

Within 4 days all symptoms had disappeared and movements of the affected joints were completely normal and painless.

Three months later blood ESR was 6 mm/hr, albumin 2.8 Gm/dl, globulin 1.8 gm/dl. He has had no recurrence of symptoms during a year follow up.

Case 8: Female, aged 29 years. Ten year history of severe rheumatoid arthritis affecting almost every joint in the body at times, but especially the left knee. She had received every form of treatment, including gold injections, penicillamine, corticosteroids and many anti-inflammatory tablets and had recently had a synovectomy of the left knee, which left it swollen and still containing large amounts of free fluid. She was confined to bed and emotionally extremely depressed.

Examination showed very active arthropathy affecting the neck, shoulders, elbows, wrists, fingers, temporomandibular joints, especially both knees with large amounts of free fluid, ankles, midtarsal and metatarsophalangeal joints. She was totally bedbound, sweating and had a temperature of 37.5-39°C. X-rays showed surprisingly little damage to cartilage and this only partial in the left knee joint. Blood showed strongly positive RF, ESR 100 mm/hr, Hb 9.8 Gm/dl, RBC 3.6 X 10^{12}/l, WBC 4.8 X 10^9/l, albumin 1.6 Gm per cent, globulin 2.8 Gm per cent.

She was treated with tinidazole 2 grams on two successive evenings followed by violent sweating, further pyrexia and increased pain and swelling of all her joints gradually dying down during the next two weeks.

Within four weeks she was able to walk and within three months apart from the operated left knee all the joints were cool, unswollen and movements normal and painless. The fluid in the left knee had absorbed, but walking was still painful to some extent.

During the next two years her life has become completely normal except for some pain in the left knee after prolonged walking. She is able to look after her house and husband and do a full time job and take a degree at the Open University. Blood count now is completely normal, ESR 4 mm/hour, RF negative, albumin 2.9 Gm/dl, globulin 1.8 Gm/dl.

She requires no further treatment.

Case 9: Girl aged 18 years, born with juvenile arthritis with marked deformities and had received prednisolone treatment almost since birth. She complained of pain in the back, in feet and hands and her growth was stunted.

On examination she showed the typical changes of Still's disease affecting the spine, wrists, fingers, knees, ankles and feet. The child was in continuous pain and tearful with severe growth stunting. Blood showed ESR 60 mm/hr, positive RF, HB 5.0/dl, RBC 2.5 X 10^{12}/l, albumin 1.2 Gm percent, globulin 3.0 Gm per cent. X-rays showed gross kyphoscoliosis of the spine and marked deformities of the wrists, fingers, ankles, feet and toes.

She was treated with one gram tinidazole on two successive evenings which produced a short lived Herxheimer reaction, but within four weeks the patient was obviously in much less pain and in two months was completely free of pain and the joint movements were markedly freer.

The prednisolone was gradually tapered off. She gradually began to grow in the next year and grew two inches in height and was able to walk about though the deformities remained. She has been able to play games with school friends and after 1-1/2 years all the blood parameters are within normal limits.

Case 10: Male aged 65 years. Slow onset of pain in the left shoulder and left side of the neck and tingling down the outside of the arm, forearm and into the fingers followed by pain and swelling of the right wrist and right index finger making work impossible.

Examination showed a painful, fixed left shoulder, tenderness on pressure over the cervical spine and pain, hotness, swelling and tenderness of all joints of the right middle finger. X-rays of the shoulders were normal, of the neck showed some degree of spondylitis and of the right middle finger were normal. Blood showed doubtful positive RF, but was otherwise normal.

He was treated with 2 grams of tinidazole on each of two successive evenings which resulted in violent night sweats and a pyrexia with further swelling of the finger.

On the third day the movements of the shoulders were completely painless and free and three weeks later the finger was completely normal.

He has remained well over the next two years and is now able to play golf.

Disease activity was assessed clinically before, during and at the end of observations. Pain and stiffness was scored subjectively according to an arbitrary scale, severe (3), moderate (2), mild (1), and absent (0).

A Ritchie articular index was used to assess joint tenderness and grip strengths were measured with a sphygmomanometer bag inflated to 30mm of mercury. Laboratory measurements included C-reactive protein by single radial immuno-defusion, immuno complexes by liquid-phase Clq-binding assay and IgM rheumatoid factor by an enzyme-linked immuno-assay and red and white blood cell counts by the standard methods. The ESR was carried out in the normal manner.

Conclusion

In all of the 10 cases tinidazole induced sweating, pyrexia and exaggeration of the symptoms of active disease both in the affected tissues and the appearance of inflammation in other joints, not previously affected. This exaggeration of symptoms is typical of an Herxheimer reaction.

These phenomena gradually settled down during the next few months and after one year joints in which no radiological damage was present were normal clinically.

The accompanying parotid swelling and ulcerative colitis

cleared permanently. In joints with erosion of cartilage or bone deformities, symptoms persisted. After a year the blood changes returned to normal.

(Based on   Archimedes A. Concon, M.D., Memphis, Tennessee)

Introduction

Dr. Archimedes A. Concon is a Memphis physician who has apparently had the experience of trying antiamoebic drugs on a wide variety of ailments. From among the variety submitted for publication the author has chosen the following, which includes the effect of metronidazole on psoriasis, lupus erythematosus, and rheumatoid arthritis, all diseases which are supposedly incurable within the present state of art of medical treatments.

Successive cases treated with metronidazole

Case 1: A 33 year old white male patient came to see me with a history of psoriasis involving the hands and fingers of 12 years duration. Patient was put on metronidazole 500 mg 4 tablets (2 Gm) after supper daily for 2 days, rest 5 days, and repeat course indefinitely until well. At end of 4 months the skin on the hands were largely clear. Most of the fingernails were normal looking. At the end of 6 months, patient was clinically free.

Case 2: A 61 year old white female patient came in with complaints of rheumatoid arthritis involving the hands, left hip, and knees of 14 years duration. She was barely able to use her hands or walk at the time I saw her because of stiffness and pain of joints involved. She was put on metronidazole 500 mg 4 tablets (2 Gm) after supper daily for 2 days, rest 5 days and repeat course indefinitely until well. At the end of 3 months from start of treatment stiffness and pain in joints were very much less. At the end of 5 months from start of treatment stiffness and pain of joints were hardly noticeable. At the end of 6 months from start of treatment, patient was clinically free. During course of treatment patient complained of chronic nausea which was bearable. The chronic nausea disappeared after termination of treatment.

Case 3: A 29 white male patient came in with a history of systemic lupus erythematosus, of 7 years duration with recent kidneys involvement. His albuminuria (urinary protein) was 2+. Urinary output was adequate, at start of treatment. Patient was put on metronidazole 500 mg 4 tablets (2 Gm) after supper daily for 2 days, rest 5 days, and repeat course indefinitely until well. After 1 month of treatment his albuminuria was 1+. His urinary output was adequate. At the end of 5 months from start of treatment his albuminuria was negative. His urinary output remained adequate. At the end of 6 months from start of treatment, his albuminuria was negative and his urinary output was adequate. Patient could tolerate exposure to sunlight where before he could not. Patient was declared clinically free.

Conclusion

The above findings apparently show that the *Limax amoeba* is responsible (as reported by Professor Roger Wyburn-Mason) for more than limited forms of rheumatoid diseases.

(Based on Robert Bingham [Report],
Desert Hot Springs, California)

Introduction

Robert Bingham, M. D., was Chief of Orthopaedic Surgery of the Surgical Section, Esperanza Inter-community Hospital, Yorba Linda, CA, and is Medical Administrator of the Desert Arthritis Medical Clinic in Desert Hot Springs, CA. He's had a special interest in arthritis for more than 30 years, which began when he was an intern at the University of Pennsylvania Hospital, and continued under several renown specialists over the years. In August 1976 Dr. Bingham visited Professor Roger Wyburn-Mason in England, and followed up the visit with the article "Rheumatoid Disease: Has One Investigator Found its Cause and Its Cure?" This is the same article credited by Jack M. Blount, M.D. in Chapter 2 which led to the vital clues that saved his life.

According to a second article[5] by Robert Bingham, the first medical information on clotrimazole to be published in Britain appeared in the *Lancet*, Feb. 28, 1976 as a medical letter from Professor Wyburn-Mason. Therein Wyburn-Mason reported the first ten patients treated whose signs and symptoms of active rheumatoid disease disappeared in from 3 to 28 days and showed no return of the disease in a one year follow-up.

In his article, Dr. Bingham describes results of over two hundred patients treated by Professor Wyburn-Mason, and includes the following case histories based on interviewing Roger Wyburn-Mason and reviewing case reports and letters from patients who had been treated with clotrimazole.

Effects of treatment with clotrimazole

Case 1: . . . He was suffering from painful and complete anklyosis of the spine and other joints of the limbs. The disease had lasted 33 years. He could not move his neck or back at all, and the joints of his extremities were swollen, tender and painful. His spine, hips and knees were flexed and fixed so that his eyes were directed toward the floor when he was standing. In 12 weeks on clotrimazole 2 gm per day he was able to move his spine almost normally and to stand erect. The swelling in his hands and feet subsided and he was able to walk with a normal gait. He is now decorating his house, digging the garden and driving an automobile again for the first time in 30 years.

Case 2: . . . .a physician's 5-year-old daughter, had very acute painful and tender joints and night sweats with elevated temperatures continually up to 106° F. She was taking prednisone 80 mg per day. Her temperature fell to normal in 12 hours after beginning clotrimazole and remained down, enabling prednisone to be stopped without return of symptoms.

67

Case 3: Another child — 13 years of age — had the disease since she was 1 year old. Symptoms included a low hemoglobin. Her spleen was huge and the sedimentation rate elevated to 60 mm/hr. Her hands, knees, ankles and feet were swollen, and she was in constant pain. She had been taking prednisone 5 mg and Indocin® 50 mg per day with only partial relief of pain. Within 2 days of clotrimazole treatment, her temperature dropped to normal for the first time in months. By the end of 3 weeks the corticosteroid and pain-relieving drugs could be stopped and she was walking comfortably. Her hemoglobin increased from 50% normal to 80% normal in just a few weeks. At the end of 12 weeks, all signs of active rheumatoid arthritis had subsided.

Case 4: . . . a boy age 5, proved that the most dramatic results with clotrimazole occur in juvenile arthritis. He was completely handicapped by pain, swelling and joint deformities from onset of the disease. He had been taking prednisone 30 mg per day. He was 9 inches too short and 20 pounds overweight for his age. In 3 or 4 days after the start of clotrimazole (500 mg once a day), he had so much relief of pain and swelling that his actions were "lively and comfortable." He became almost uncontrollable . . . The cortisone was decreased at the rate of 5 mg each week, and he continued to improve. Clotrimazole was given at 500 mg/day for 5 weeks and then decreased to 250 mg/day for 7 more weeks. After 12 weeks, it appeared that he had made a "full recovery." After a year he has remained well and is now of normal weight and height for his age.

The Treatment of Rheumatoid Disease With Anti-protozoal Drugs

A Preliminary Report By Robert Bingham, M.D.

On a clinical basis . . . treatment of rheumatoid arthritis and its related forms of disease with anti-protozoal drugs has proven very successful. This infectious origin of rheumatoid arthritis explains the success in the use of chloroquine which has anti-protozoal properties as well as anti-malarial action.

Over the last six years our clinic has used various anti-protozoal drugs for the treatment of active rheumatoid arthritis in over 500 cases. We have not done double-blind placebo studies for lack of research funding. However, we have used two groups of patients, one not treated at all, the second group treated by conventional methods such as with gold, penicillamine, and anti-inflammatory drugs, and we have compared our results with six medications which have anti-protozoal properties.

Dr. Roger Wyburn-Mason recommends tinidazole (Fasigyn®) which is available in Great Britain but not in the United States. He believes it is more effective and has less side-effects than any of the drugs used in this study. We have found di-hydroxyquin (Diodoquin®) and metronidazole (Flagyl®) to be very effective and adequate in our series. If a patient shows any side-effects to one of these, such as nausea or loss of appetite, or if the particular case shows some resistance to treatment then a change to the other of these two drugs has often been effective in relieving the patients acute symptoms. The failure rate of patients with active rheumatoid arthritis treated with anti-protozoal drugs has been about 6%.

Flagyl® (metronidazole) is given as follows: for a 150 pound male (70) kg.), three tablets of 250 mg. each three times a day for ten days, a total of ninety tablets. With women patients weighing approximately 120 pounds (50 kg.), two tablets of 250 mg. three times a day for ten days, a total of sixty tablets. Then the medicine is stopped from one to five months. If there is a recurrence of symptoms or a continued activity then the medicine is repeated for three days, one tablet (250 mg.) three times a day, a total of nine tablets.

In using Diodoquin® (di-iodohydroxiquin), the dosage is two tablets (650) mg. per tablet), three times a day for ten days, a total of sixty tablets. If the medicine has to be repeated in one to five months then one tablet is given three times a day for 3 days, a total of nine tablets. These medications should be given with food or milk, preferably at the beginning or in the middle of a meal. Except for occasional nausea or anorexia, we have found no side-effects. We have had no drug reactions or complications with these medicines in the dosages mentioned.
. . . . . .

Results: 500 patients have been treated with anti-protozoal drugs. All had active rheumatoid arthritis with elevated sedimentation rates and positive rheumatoid serology. Of these, 278 patients showed improvement, 137 showed complete remissions and 85 had no improvement with the first drug used, 30 of these responded to the second course of treatment or the second drug used.

Comparative Results of Treatment With Other Drugs

	Patients Treated	Improved or Remissions	%Change
Controls	22	7	30
Conventional Care	30	8	27
Copper Sulfate	12	8	66
Bile Salts	12	9	75
Clotrimazole	9	7	78
Diodoquin®	204	189	93
Chloroquine	12	6	50
Flagyl®	221	181	82*

* *Recent cases have done better on increased dosages.*

Conclusions

The discovery of Dr. Roger Wyburn-Mason that many cases of rheumatoid arthritis are infectious origin with either amoeba *Limax* or ameoba *Naegleria* seems confirmed by success with treatment of acute active cases using anti-protozoal drugs. Diodoquin® and Flagyl® have been the most successful. Further clinical and pathological studies are recommended to verify these results and determine the pathological relationships between the protozoa and the rheumatoid diseases.

Conclusion

Apparently there is a wide range of antiamoebics that will kill the *Limax amoeba.* Clotrimazole was one of the very first, and it was no less effective than those that are in general use now.

[1] Gunby, P. "Allopurinol Treatment for Protozoal Infections", *J. Amer. Med. Ass.*, 1978, Medical News, 1941-2, p. 240.

[2] Wyburn-Mason, Roger, *The Causation of Rheumatoid Disease and Many Human Cancers — A New Concept in Medicine*, Iji Publishing Co., Ltd., Tokyo, Japan.

[3] Wyburn-Mason, Roger, "The Naeglerial Causation of Rheumatoid and Many Human Cancers. A New Concept in Medicine," *Medical Hypotheses*, 5: 1237-1249, 1979.

[4] Wojtulewski, J.A., et. al., *Annals of the Rheumatic Disease*, 39, 469-472, 1980.

⁵ *Orthopaedic Review*, "Dr. Roger Wyburn-Mason Is Alive and Back at Work, The Protozoal Theory of Rheumatoid Disease, A Progress Report and a Drug for Treating It", Robert Bingham, M.D., 1977, pp. 23-26.

Irony

In America much is made out of the idea of double-blind experiments, which are quite costly, and perhaps can help discriminate between one aspirin substitute and another. Rheumatologists have insisted on double-blind experiments which are supposed to be the ultimate in "scientific" proof, — although their own routine usage of gold shots and penicillamine have no scientific basis — the lack of such studies kept Wyburn-Mason's findings from the general public for six years.

According to my recent letter, "Roger Wyburn-Mason told the story of his student who orignially wrote up the double-blind trial method in the *Lancet* and the Editor gave a glowing appraisal of the method. It was then seized on as the perfect proof of all new therapies and was adopted. The first one done was on the use of Cortisone in Asthma and the result of this trial was that it showed quite conclusively that Cortisone has no effect on Asthma! It is well known that the most effective therapy for asthma is Cortisone. So where do we go from here?"

[Name witheld by author]

"Chance only favours the mind that is prepared." — Louis Pasteur.

ROGER WYBURN-MASON

Letter received, May 1983

Many substances having in common the fact that they kill free-living amoebae have been found when administered to sufferers from active rheumatoid disease to cause a transient but rapid increase in the symptoms of the latter followed by marked improvement or complete disappearance of disability and pain. Deformities are, however, not usually affected. These substances have no effect in healthy subjects. Because of this property of first increasing the symptoms of the disease before lessening or abolishing them it is impossible to carry out a double blind trial with them on rheumatoid patients. Rheumatologists have seized on this as a reason for not accepting the idea that these drugs are of benefit to such patients, whereas, in fact, if given correctly they invariably cause the activity of the disease to cease and in early cases result in complete cure. Rheumatologists refuse to try the treatment on patients to see if they get similar results, which is the true test of a scientific discovery. Instead unscientifically they dismiss anti-amoebic treatment out of hand simply because no double blind trial has been carried out owing to the impossibility of doing them. They ignore the fact that if a substance has already been found to be curative then no double blind trial is necessary. None was carried out in humans in proving the benefit of salvarsan in cases of syphilis, of the original sulphonamides in many human bacterial infections [Professor Roger Wyburn-Mason took part in the original trials of sulphonamides], or the first human trials of penicillin on infections.

Eminent [ethical] doctors maintain that once a drug treatment has been shown to be superior in treating any disease other drugs should be abandoned. This applies to rheumatoid disease when the pain and suffering can be rapidly brought to a halt with the giving of anti-amoebic drugs. Only this group of drugs should be continued to be used in the treatment of rheumatoid disease. Failure to do so could be unethical and amount to malpractice or negligence.

71

Chapter IX
Correspondence, Testimonials, and Book Report
From Dr. Paul K. Pybus[1],
Pietermaritzburg, South Africa

(To *The Beebe News*, Beebe, Arkansas) "Other doctors in South Africa are also using metronidazole with equally good results. It really works. I also know Professor Wyburn-Mason who first advised its use to me. Many years ago I was his House Physician.

"Doctor Blount is doing wonderful work . . . . The whole world must know what has been discovered. . . ."

(To Dr. Jack M. Blount) ". . . one must promote a cure if we have one. If the medical profession will not accept it then it must be stated elsewhere. Neither of us wish to keep our secrets for our own monetary gain. The Hippocratic oath tells us to teach our colleagues. If any doctor is man enough, and there are many of them, to bring a patient to me I will not only treat the patient but give the doctor details of how to do it. I have myself not only done this but also even given the doctor materials with which I work. My methods are open for all to see and for those who wish to learn so that all may benefit. I know that yours are also."

From Bob Kemp, Beebe, Arkansas

(From Bob Kemp, editor of The Beebe News, Beebe, Arkansas) "I took the first dose of Flagyl at 5 p.m. on Thursday, Oct. 29. Eight tablets, 250 milligrams each, were swallowed following a supper meal. Two hours earlier — at about 3 p.m. — I took a 400 milligram Motrin tablet, a medication which had been in use several months. This was the final Motrin tablet. Within just a few hours — before bedtime — I began experiencing less pain.

"During the early morning hours — some 7 hours after the initial Flagyl dosage — a headache developed, but nothing else. The patient took three aspirin tablets, went back to bed and the headache quit. Less and less body pain was experienced Friday morning and a previously severe pain in the right knee — the most troublesome pain in the past — was completely gone. This remains so at the writing of these comments on Tuesday morning. The second dose of Flaygl — another 2,000 milligrams or 2 grams — was taken at 4 p.m. Friday. This dose — taken on a partially empty stomach, not recommended by Dr. Blount — produced nausea but not severe enough to vomit. Also a headache developed a few hours after the second dose. Three aspirin tablets (5 grains each) ended the headache rather quickly. On arising from bed Saturday morning, all arthritic pain — and all other pain — had vanished. It seemed like a miracle had happened. This general feeling of well-being continues."

(Reprint from *The Beebe News*, Beebe, Arkansas) On Wednesday, Nov. 25, Dr. Blount flew to Chattanooga, TN, to appear on a morning television show on Channel 12, with the show host: Harry Thornton, and a woman colleague.

Several of Dr. Blount's patients from the Chattanooga area were at the studio to give results of his treatment. What they said was almost unbelievable. Dr. Blount provided *The Beebe News* with an audio tape of the program. The following information is from that audio tape:

A woman that identified herself as Louise Searcy said:

"I was almost in a wheel chair. I was just dragging my feet and could not hardly go any steps or anything. And I went down there to Philadelphia, [Mississippi] that

73

morning and got up the next morning after driving and I was almost crying with my knees hurting me so bad. On the way home they relieved me. After my first treatment I felt better all the way home. That was the first day of October. I'm doing square dancing now."

And the woman invited the TV audience to come and see her square dance at a nearby center that day.

A man who identified himself as W.M. Hill gave this account:

"I had osteoarthritis. Not the crippling kind. I've had it 36 years, 6 months and 6 days before going to Dr. Blount. I took so much pain pills in those amount of years that I came up with heart trouble. But I haven't had any pain since I left Dr. Blount's office at Philadelphia two weeks ago today. I haven't took any pain killers since then and haven't needed any pain killers. I was living off pain killers. I was living off pain killers for 36 years, 6 months and 6 days."

Others in the studio audience gave testimonials of benefits and the TV hosts told of hearing similar glowing reports from other persons in the area. A woman who said she is Helen Erwin told of breaking-out and having some swelling after her first dose of Flagyl. She commented that the druggist, because of this, would not refill her Flagyl prescription.

Dr. Blount commented: "The druggist was right in not refilling the prescription *under the circumstances.*" But Dr. Blount explained that such reaction "does happen — even though it is rare." However, he told the woman that a short course of cortisone-like injections (Depo Medrol) "usually takes care of that all right." "Most such patients," he said, "are able to take the medicine (Flagyl) eventually."

At this point in the TV show, Dr. Blount was told by the TV Woman Hostess: "I have talked to people who have gone down to see you who were just about carried into your office and by the time they got back to Chattanooga, they were walking and doing well."

TV Host Thornton commented: "Dr. Blount, do you feel your treatment is a cure for arthritis or just a pain reliever? Replied Dr. Blount: "I think it is a cure." Dr. Blount explained that the patient's diagnosis has to be right.

"I have had patients brought in with broken hips and told at the door they have arthritis."

"Can the treatment do anything about deformity?"

"Not much," answered Dr. Blount.

Dr. Blount was asked what percentage of success had he accomplished in arthritis: "Almost universal," was his reply.

A TV studio question to Dr. Blount by a TV watcher asked: "Do you treat arthritis and bursitis the same way?"

"We treat them the same. It is the same germ that is the troublemaker," said Dr. Blount.

"Is the Flagyl treatment employed by you for fibrositis?"

"It is" said Dr. Blount.

"Can a person with a heart condition or a diabetic take this treatment?"

"Yes, Sir. Many such are taking it already."

Regarding bachaches and those who have had back surgery: "We treat those people." Dr. Blount explained that if the original cause was the germ, the germ is still there after the operation and in those cases Flagyl is the treatment that he has found effective.

"We treat those people and they get well of their backaches . . . . even those who have had several operations on their backs."

Asked about gout, Dr. Blount said that condition is caused by buildup of uric acid caused by faulty metabolism. Flagyl, he said, is not the treatment for gout.

"One reason I am here is to tell people who have arthritis that there *is* hope. Up until now they have been told there is nothing that can be done constructively about it. But to say there is no hope to a patient, *that is hell.* There is hope. Almost all can improve. New cases can get well," declared Dr. Blount.

During the TV appearance, Dr. Blount was told by the TV Woman Reporter: "I know of people who could not do their own work or comb their own hair. They are now doing their own work . . . and this just a week later after treatment."

The TV Hostess further commented on Dr. Blount's remarkable results.

"That's a gift of God," commented Dr. Blount.

"What has been the reaction of organized medicine?"

"It has been hard for them to accept it right now, because they have been taught the orthodox, and fear of litigation . . . and errors," replied Dr. Blount.

"A gift of God we cannot hide. We must pass it on," commented the TV Woman Hostess.

"Right," said Dr. Blount.

In closing the TV program, TV Host Thornton gave these kind words to Dr. Blount: "I wish I could say how much I appreciate this man. Coming at his own expense, getting a plane, having a pilot with him and flying up here. I wish I could say how much I appreciate him going to all that trouble and expense. He did it because of his interest in reaching people and helping people. I just wish we covered the entire United States, so the people everywhere might know that there is hope for them."

From A.W. Hamilton[2], Salisbury, Rhodesia

(To Dr. John R.A. Simoons) "It seems to me that Roger Wyburn-Mason has been the first man to make a positive suggestion in the cause and the treatment of rheumatoid arthritis. The announcement appeared remotely in one of our Rhodesian papers, and my wife latched on to it smartly. We lost no time and I simply wrote to Wyburn-Mason.

"Fan me with a plate of soup if I don't get a reply by return of post.

"My own case history goes back over 16 years, and I can genuinely trace it to a fall on the polo field at the time, complicated by an onset of 'Tick-bite fever'. The name of the fever may, in fact, be a bit of a misnomer. Suffice it to say that the fever ran to a very high temperature, days in bed, and profuse sweating.

"Subsequently my left knee began to swell, and cartilage trouble was diagnosed. Out came one cartilage. No improvement whatsover. The following year, a second surgeon diagnosed the trouble as coming from my groin and wanted to operate. I put a stop to that, smartly. On the third year, the inner cartilage was removed with much ado. No improvement whatsoever, although I was beginning to know the nurses by their first names. It's an ill wind . . . .

"Tiring of the sight of knives and hospital food in Rhodesia, I took myself off to Scotland in the hope that, if the worst came to worst, I could die on my native soil. With the abandon which comes from experience, I stuck myself into the Royal Infirmary in Glasgow, under Professor Watson-Buchanan, head of arthritic research at the Royal Infirmary. Three months and 36 X-rays later, I am advised by Professor Watson-Buchanon that I have nothing more romantic than Rheumatoid Arthritis. Steroids and aspirin until the end of my days were prescribed. I prescribed for 12 further pain-racked years.

"In the interval, the R.A. seemed to spread, first to my toes, then to the other knee, and, as you know, I've only got two, my thumbs and my right shoulder. By this stage I began to look like a cross between a mouse with dysentery, and a camel with glandular fever.

"I spent my time going about saying . . . 'Oh, Death, where is they sting'.

"Enter the article by Dr. Wyburn-Mason.

75

"Mind you, in the interval I had been cheered. I had been cheered by people reminding me of the man who had NO legs.

"Orthodox medicine seemed to have failed. In Africa I had an alternative which I even considered. A witch Doctor! Certain it was that his results could not have been less negative. However, I am a bit scared of witch Doctors in case they ask me to eat my young. I did not want to commit three gorgeous daughters to the frying pan. One daughter, incidentally, having spent a year in Hollywood [California], a fully qualified nursing sister, looking after the brat of. . . . It should have been me. . . .

"Cautiously I hoped that Wyburn-Mason might JUST have the answer. An arthritic ship will, perforce, seek any port in a storm.

"The books . . . *There IS a cure for Arthritis, Arthritis and Common Sense*, . . . line my shelves. I must consign them to the flame and the lazy. Boiled elephant dung has even been suggested. I have been trying for some time to catch an elephant. They are non-cooperative. In addition, I do not run fast enough.

"Little is left, except Wyburn-Mason. It made sense. A bug, eating away at the tissues between the joints, bone against bone, distortion and infinite pain. Let's have a crack at Doc. Roger.

"With all the will in the world it is difficult to sit down, when invited, on a seat laced with a pin. Remove the pin and I shall be happy to sit down. Thus it was with the 'experts' screaming at me to keep movement going. Remove the pin, or the pain, and I'll sit down happily. None had removed the pin.

"I must correct you here. After 14 days I began to FEEL that something was happening with clotrimazole. After 16 years, there seems little hope for the apparently hopelessly distorted joints from assuming the appearance of those given to a new born babe, but hope does still spring Eternal after clotrimazole. In the event, I was able to get off steroids for the first time in 11 years, and the masses of aspirin with which I alternated, — up to 15 aspirin per day at times.

"Now, weather does seem to have an effect, and if it is cold and wet, Bob's-your-Uncle, pain. Diet too, I consider most important, without being a faddist. . . . After 7 years of being denied the fairways, I am back on the links, not yet down to the old scratch golf standard, but shaping. When I re-started last year, the Captain of the local golf club picked me out for playing the ball from the Ladies' tee. I told him to get out of my road and let me hit my third shot.

. . . .

"The degree of morning stiffness has been improved by, I would say, 75%.

"All in all, I personally feel, after 16 odd years, that Wyburn-Mason HAS found the answer and daily my mobility is improved. However, now in my fifties, do not expect me to break any track records, play golf again for the Royal Air Force, or play polo for Rhodesia."

From E. H. C., Ph.D., Chevy Chase, MD

(To John R.A. Simoons, 1979)"I am a male, 67, who still likes to engage in vigorous physical activities. I was under treatment by Dr. _____ for chronic rheumatoid arthritis from late in 1973 or early 1974 until January 1977.

"My medical history indicates I showed evidence of the infection prior to 1974: Various forms of bursitis (1961-1973), gout (1964) and periodontal disease (1971).

"Aside from aspirin, the drugs which Dr. _____ prescribed were Motrin® and Tandearil® (1974-5), Indocin®, Ilosone®, Naprosyn®, Butzoladin® and Tolectin® in 1976. (Tolectin gave me the most unpleasant side reactions I ever had from a drug.) I was given Plaquenil® in 1976 and 1977. In addition, when the pains were too great, Dr. _____ injected cortisone in the knees. There was never any improvement and indeed I fully expected to be crippled. I gave up almost all exercise and sports; even stair climbing often required going up on hands and knees.

"The 1975 report on rheumatoid arthritis, and its successful cure, by Prof. Roger Wyburn-Mason to the International Conference on Chemotherapy in London received extensive but garbled coverage in the *Washington Star*. This I clipped for reference. In 1976 the National Institute of Arthritis published *How to Cope with Arthritis* which stated that neither the cause of nor a cure for arthritis was known. This was confirmed by other authoritative sources. It was obvious I was spending a great deal of money with no hope for improvement.

"When my wife and I went to Switzerland in the winter of 1977 I flew to London to see Wyburn-Mason. I saw him again before we left Switzerland. I have had his constant advice and assistance since that time.

"On my first visit he gave me an imidazole compound not otherwise identified. I was scarce prepared, back in Switzerland, for the violence of the reaction and pain which I began to experience some 46 hours after taking the first dose. It reached over a period of days to every part of my body below the neck. It was almost like a lesson in anatomy and physiology as the stabbing pains spread; they confirmed Prof. Wyburn-Mason's statement that the infection was universal in my body. The second dose of tablets produced nearly as strong a reaction. Thereafter the pains became less intense. When I went again to London I was told to take imidazole tablets only when the preceding pain had virtually disappeared.

"In May 1977 I attended a dance where, without thinking about it, I was on the floor for three hours. This was the point where I realized how effective the antiprotozoal drugs had been. I subsequently and quickly returned to tennis, squash, golf, swimming, etc. There was a noticeable change in my appearance, remarked upon by many people to my wife. Rheumatoid disease is depressing and debilitating, as well as painful.

"I had not informed my Washington physician of my new treatment, prior to going to London, since Prof. Wyburn-Mason could give me no advance assurance of success. Some time later when I was sure the treatment had worked, I sent him a written report. In September and October 1977 he gave me a complete physical, with further checkups thereafter. He found no trace of rheumatic pains in any of the joints, which he had unsuccessfully treated for several years previously. My RF was negative; my ESR which was 40mms per hour soon dropped to 30. It has not been checked since that time. Dr. _____ was sufficiently impressed with the results to phone them to Dr. _____, a leading Washington-area rheumatologist. The latter asked me for a sample of the drugs to analyze. I have heard nothing further on this. Subsequently I lent Prof. Wyburn-Mason's book to Dr. _____. Prof. Wyburn-Mason later assured me my ESR was not unusually high after a course of potent antiprotozoan drugs.

"In September 1977 Prof. Wyburn-Mason provided me, through a friend, a supply of tinidazole tablets from Switzerland. Although I had no arthritic pain, I still had lingering reactions to the drugs, indicating I might still have some limax amebae in the system. In the winter of 1977-78, when I was again in Switzerland and Italy, I replenished, with Prof. Wyburn-Mason's prescription, the supply of tinidazole and added Naxogin®. I was advised to continue to use them from time to time as a safeguard. By then I had little or no reaction to the drugs. Although I felt I should not resume alpine skiing, I was able to take lessons in Swiss cross-country skiing, which is a vigorous enough exercise."

The insidious nature of reinfection is shown by the follow-up letter received recently (1982) by the author from E. H. C., Ph.D.:

"I have had, since then, serious relapses, as I seem to be genetically highly sensitive to the amoeba involved. Most likely I was being reinfected by our swimming pool which we keep heated all winter. After conferring with Prof. Wyburn-Mason, I have now added copper plates and copper sulphate to the pool, to kill the infective organisms.

"I have also been under an intensive course of treatments, this winter and spring, with allopurinol, felden, and furaxolidone. I am greatly improved but I cannot yet say I have had a complete cure."

On making further queries of Professor Wyburn-Mason regarding a situation in Tennessee (USA), where perhaps eighty percent of the well and spring water contains coliform bacteria — implying that the protozoa must also be present — the Professor replied as follows:

"As regards sterilizing of your water supply — the protozoon is killed not only by copper sulphate, but also by metallic copper[3], but not by chlorine. The simplest way to get over the problem of the organism in the drinking water is to have pipes from the reservoir changed to copper ones. However, while you can take reasonable precautions not to take the organism into the body, one is always left with the fact that the cysts float in the air and can be taken in by breathing or talking. There is no way of preventing this unless you are one of the lucky ones and the organisms you inhale are not pathogenic."

Interviews

The author interviewed patients as they entered Dr. Blount's office, finding that most were there, from scattered parts of the country, because of what they had seen happen to friends, neighbors, and relatives. . . . Their responses were overwhelmingly enthusiastic. They told of those they'd personally witnessed, who'd not been able to work, or to walk, or were suffering considerably, and now could work, or walk, or were free of pain. The author, of course, could not collect statistics on such short notice; and, in any case, such numbers would not have satisfied the more stringent requirements of scientific "double-blind" experiments. Nonetheless, having had personal experience with the antiamoebic treatment, having read Professor Roger Wyburn-Mason's technical research findings, having interviewed patients — and having had some technical knowledge of bio-statistical requirements — its problems and pitfalls — there was little the author could do but be impressed.

Letters to and on File with Dr. Jack M. Blount

(From Mrs. A.B.M., Chattanooga, Tennessee) "Just a note to let you know how we are feeling. Mrs. G. is better than she has been in over *6 years.* She is having *no pains hardly*, and planning a trip to New Orleans to visit her grand-daughter, when she hasn't been able to even go to the grocery store. She's driving her car, going where she needs to go now. My sister, M.H., was feeling much better while she was at my apartment, but she left on Wednesday after we were to see you on a Monday. She was awful sick vomiting. She said her stomach was full of gas, and she was so sick, but I haven't heard anything else. Myself I feel much better. I think the treatment has helped my headaches as much as my arthritis pains. My pains in my fingers I still have. I have a breaking out on my bottom, but I don't believe the medicine I am taking has anything to do with it. Enjoyed your appearance on H's show and it was nice seeing you again."

(From Mrs. E.K., Trenton, Tennessee) "I was in your office Thursday of last week. I began my medicine on Friday. Today I am free of pain for the first time. I really feel as if I want to do things, and to go somewhere. It is unbelievable."

(From B.D., Killen, Alabama) "I am writing you to let you know that my father is doing great since he seen you the 23rd of November. He has not missed any work and is dressing himself now. We all want to thank you so much."

(From E. H., Florence, Alabama) "Hello
"I am feeling fine. Thanks to Dr. Blount."

(From A.S.B., Rogersville, Alabama) "I am sure you will be glad to know that I am doing very well following my visit and treatment.
"I was down there December 18, 1981.
"I finished my medication two weeks ago. The last two weeks of Flagyl made me feel sick to the stomach but vomited only twice.
"Some mornings I feel a little stiff but the severe pain is gone. Sometimes I feel a weakness in the lower back but not the pain I once had. Other joints of the body have some soreness but very little."

(From G.H., Savannah, Tennessee) "I was down there and had a treatment October 26. I have not had a pain since. Since I was there it has helped my husband and Mrs. W. too. . . . I think you will be getting some calls from Savannah for treatments as I am just fine."

(From an English physician who prefers to remain anonymous; [*Note that this physician had been corresponding with Dr. Jack M. Blount from time to time and especially arguing that Dr. Blount could not help the long-term arthritic in the manner reported, and that he, personally, had not seen the same results from such patients that Dr. Jack Blount had reported*]) "He was a 63 year old man from Georgia, USA, who insisted on coming to see me although I tried to advise him that he was really so bad it would be a waste of time. He was the worst case of rheumatoid arthritis I had ever seen. Every joint in his body, including cryo-arytenoids, was completely ankylosed. He could only speak in a whisper, could not move his bowed head and was brought in in a wheel chair. I treated him much against my will because I thought he would be wasting his time and money, but he implored me to do so as I was his last hope. He had travelled all over the world including going to Taiwan for acupuncture. Curiously his condition was quite painless, since all joint movement was prevented by adhesions. The disease had begun 33 years before at which time he had had to give up driving his car. I gave him metronidazole at four weekly intervals. He had only a mild Jarisch-Herxheimer reaction, but then the most astonishing things began to happen. Normally his wife used to put him to bed and he lay on one side quite immovable until she turned him in the middle of the night. About five days after the first dose of tablets, while lying in bed he suddenly threw his right arm out and found he could extend it fully at the elbow after a loud cracking of the adhesions. This process went on over the next few months and five months after returning to the USA he wrote to me in his own hand (previously impossible) to say that he was now symptomless, had just dug his garden, planted flowers, painted and decorated his house inside and out, bought a new car and he and his wife were going for their first holiday in 33 years. This is a remarkable case."

Book Report by Dr. Robert Bingham[4]

Each generation of man develops a few independent medical investigators whose recognition may be long delayed. This is true as well of the inventors, geniuses, and original thinkers in other fields. But confirmation and proof of a discovery in medicine may be controversial for many years.

This may be the fate of the author of this new book by Professor Roger Wyburn-Mason. He has for more than twenty years researched the roles of pathogenic protozoa in human diseases. For twelve years he has been writing a monumental work, in collaboration with his wife, which may revolutionize the diagnosis and treatment of many chronic and dangerous illnesses.

After taking his degrees at Christ's College, Cambridge, England, where he was also a Fellow, he was an associate professor and lecturer at Yale in the United States. He then returned to London as a research fellow in Royal Marsden Hospital, London, Prophit Research, in microbiology.

While serving as a physician in the Ealing-Hammersmith and Hounslow Health Authority hospitals and laboratories he discovered pathogenic protozoa in arthritis patients from all tissues of the body. He was amazed to find these in cases of rheumatoid arthritis and in some forms of cancer and degenerative diseases — all conditions considered by most doctors to be of "unknown etiology" and generally incurable as well.

The Preface states: "What is required in the search for the causes of rheumatoid disease and human cancer are not just increasing expenditures of money for traditional research but new ideas. This book puts forward such new ideas and shows how clinically and pathologically they fit the known facts about both rheumatoid disease and many cases of human cancer."

He discovered that the organisms responsible for rheumatoid arthritis are *limax amoebae*. They are found in brackish waters and affect certain susceptible individuals, migrating from the gastrointestinal tract into the blood and then into the joints and other body tissues.

These are thermotrophic, or "heat-seeking," organisms and can be isolated by chilling the laboratory specimen, whereby the amoeba migrate through a fine membrane into warmed saline solution where they can be identified.

His next problem led to exploration and experimentation to find chemicals and drugs which would destroy these amoebae and control these diseases.

Several chemical compounds have proved useful, as he announced in July 1975 at the International Congress of Chemotherapy in London. One was *clotrimazole*, manufactured by Bayer in Germany. It is now undergoing further clinical tests in Germany and England and has been tested at the National Arthritis [now Desert] Medical Clinic in California.

Professor Wyburn-Mason further writes: "It seems highly probable that various species of free-living limax amoebae are the etiological agents of collagen-auto-immune diseases. In general these diseases show every gradation and combination with one another. They are not due to a single organism but to a number of similar organisms. Such a parasitic infection would explain the urticaria, asthma [intrinsic], and eosinophilia observed in many cases of collagen or auto-immune diseases.

"The failure to find such organisms in ordinary sections of tissue is due to the fact that they appear like macrophanges. They may be shown up, however, by immunofluorescent techniques."

This list of chronic and degenerative diseases, in which pathogenic protozoa have been found by Professor Wyburn-Mason and the investigators who have been studying his work, reads like a list of the unknown maladies of mankind: Paget's disease of bone, ulcerative colitis, myasthenia gravis, arteritis, chronic pyelonephritis, some cases of diabetes, pericarditis, some cases of hepatitis and cirrhosis of the liver, uterine fibroids, ovarian cysts, and in some types of malignancies such as lymphoma, leukemia and Hodgkins disease. These organisms may also cause scleroderma, alopecia, vitiligo, melanoderma, eczema, psoriasis and dermatitis herpetiformis of the skin. In the mouth they are associated with gingivitis, pyorrhea and dental caries may occur. Asthma and chronic bronchitis may appear in the lungs. Parkinson's disease of the central nervous system, psychoses, and gliomas may result from such protozoal infections[5].

They may cause many pre-malignant conditions and thus play a role in causing many human malignancies. Severe physical and nervous stress, injuries and other illnesses may precipitate these diseases by lowering local and general tissue resistance and permit the spread or localization of protozoa which under other circumstances might not cause symptoms.

Adequate Treatment[6] by Dr. Robert Bingham

A young woman patient with an early case of rheumatoid arthritis presented herself at the National [now Desert] Arthritis Medical Clinic in Desert Hot Springs for treatment. She brought with her a five-page consultation from a famous medical center. It was well written, contained an excellent medical history, a complete physical examination, many x-ray reports, and three pages of laboratory tests. The clinical diagnosis was correct: "active rheumatoid arthritis." But the treatment of her disease had failed completely. Her physician, a well-known rheumatologist, had advised her as follows: *"You have an active case of rheumatoid arthritis. I don't know whether it will get better, get worse, or become chronic. Take twelve asspirin tablets a day. Come to see me again in three months' time."* She had not improved on the "aspirin alone" therapy.

(This is not an isolated example. It is wrong only because it is inadequate. Aspirin relieves pain. It causes an increased flow of blood to the joints and has some anti-inflammatory effect. The omission of other medical advice regarding her health, diet, rest, exercise, physical therapy and vitamins handicapped her in making any improvement or recovery.)

Further evaluation of this patient showed that she was in a high stress occupation, teaching school in a neighborhood where disciplinary problems were almost out of hand, leaving her exhausted at night. She smoked too many cigarettes. She didn't get enough sleep. She was "dieting" to avoid getting fat. She was not taking any regular exercises. Her arthritis was worsening, and her impending mental and physical breakdown was feared by the school principal. He gave her a month's "sick leave." She came to the desert to recuperate in a change of environment and the dry warm desert climate. Fortunately, she had not been started on corticosteroid drugs or gold therapy. Her arthritis was early and acute and limited mostly to the metacarpal-phalangeal and proximal interphalangeal joints of her hands and feet and her wrists and elbows and knees. These joints were hot, tender, swollen and painful. On twelve aspirin a day she was capable of walking and of self care, but she had been getting worse during the past few months.

In reviewing her x-ray and laboratory findings I found a sedimentation rate of 56, a positive rheumatoid arthritis factor in the latex fixation test, a positive C-reactive protein test, a white blood count elevation of 11,000 with a slight shift to the left and 5% eosinophils. Her other blood chemistries, serological tests and urine findings were normal.

A dietary analysis was obtained, typical of one week's meals prior to her coming to the desert. This showed an inadequate protein intake for her height, weight, age, sex and physical activity. It was only 62% of normal. Her fat intake surprised her very much, because she was dieting to lose weight. It was 120% of normal. Her caloric intake was 80% of normal. She was deficient in every single vitamin and mineral. Her acid base balance was strongly to the acid side.

Since she is somewhat typical of the rheumatoid patients which we examined and treated during the past year, I will mention the features of her care.

1. She was placed on a *high protein, high vitamin diet* eliminating refined carbohydrate, high fat, processed and preserved foods. An important part of this diet is certified raw milk, fresh fruit, fresh vegetables and emphasis on nuts and grains.

2. Vitamin supplements were used therapeutically, giving her about four times the minimum daily requirements to build her vitamin reserves and improve her metabolism.
3. A hair analysis showed mineral deficiencies which were treated with chelated minerals, especially chelated magnesium.
4. She was given *"Yucca extract"* tablets as a food supplement to correct any lower bowel malfunctions and to help relieve her arthritis symptoms.
5. She was started on the *arthritis vaccine* program.
6. Female *hormones* were given first by injection, later by mouth.
7. *Physical therapy* was started, hot wax baths for her hands and wrists, and hot packs and ultrasound for her knees.
8. She took deep hot *natural mineral water therapy* two or three times a day in the pools of the motel in which she stayed in Desert Hot Springs.
9. She started a gradual program of *sunbathing* and light tanning.
10. *Exercise* was started by swimming twice a day and short walks of gradually increasing distance.
11. She was started on one of the new *anti-protozoal drugs* (Flagyl®) for a three-week period of medical care, gradually reducing her aspirin intake from forty to about ten grains a day.

This might be called an "eleven point program" for the treatment of rheumatoid arthritis.

On this regime, by the end of only four weeks, she was greatly improved. All heat and swelling had disappeared from her joints. Stiffness and limitation of motion was greatly reduced. The constant pain was relieved, permitting her to sleep without drugs. Fortunately, she had an early and fairly mild case of the disease. By six months, a follow-up examination revealed only a slight amount of stiffness in her wrists. She was considered to be "recovered" without significant permanent joint damage.

(From Terry Crommelin, Perth, Western Australia to the Author) "Perhaps you are aware of the fact that one of my close friends on holiday in America saw Dr. Robert Bingham's article at the same time as Dr. Jack M. Blount did. I immediately telephoned Dr. Bingham, recalling his amazement on hearing someone from Perth, as he passed through here during the war for one day. His words were 'By all means bring your daughter Jenny to see me, but I am not the number one man. I have commenced practicing the works of Roger Wyburn-Mason'. His charming wife respected the long distance call advising me that Professor Wyburn-Mason was recovering from a heart attack, but would speak to me.

It is history that I visited him a month or so later and arranged for my wife and my 13 year old daughter to go to London for treatment. She started on clotrimazole, then moved to Flagyl. She had been on cortisone for 10 years or more. She is now 19 years old, only 4'8" high and weighs approximately 32 kg and has recently been diagnosed as a coeliac, as my 23 year old daughter is also.

The genetic history of our family was of great interest to Professor Wyburn-Mason, particularly my wife's father being diabetic and her mother suffering from rheumatoid arthritis. The genetic build-up of the family has affected the three living children. One died after birth. Whilst crippled, Jenny has no joint pain. She takes Fasigyn regularly in small doses.

My friends with minor joint aches and pains that disturb their golf and gardening take Fasigyn with immediate results, usually four tablets every six months."

Letter by Dr. Jack M. Blount
(To Professor Wyburn-Mason) The practice of medicine is much more rewarding and satisfying since your wonderful revelations. I used to dread seeing people with rheumatoid — collagen — auto-immune — disease. I had nothing that would help appreciably. Now its a pleasure to see them. The thrill really comes when they return and tell how grateful they are that they have finally found something that really helps.

I have continued to refine and simplify the treatment. . . .

MORE LETTERS

Between the first and second editions of this book, more success letters have been received from patients and physicians, world-wide. I wanted very much to include all of them in this second edition, especially those heart-rending successes from Dr. Paul K. Pybus of Republic of South Africa.

Unfortunately, space and time preclude satisfaction of my desires; also it is unlikely that either physicians or the afflicted will be convinced by several tons of testimonials and letters — only by trying it, and observing successful results will complete acceptance of *The Rheumatoid Disease Foundation* protocol be accepted everywhere.

Dr. Paul K. Pybus has contributed in other ways most significantly to the solution of the residual pains of rheumatoid disease, known as pains of sciatica, and also in giving us an approach to handling osteoarthritis — and for that important, precious knowledge, additional book space is indeed devoted, and presented beginning page 100.

---

[1] Also see "Metronidazole in rheumatoid arthritis" **To the Editor:** *Sa Mediese Tydskrif*, 20 Februarie 1982, pp. 261-2, P.K. Pybus, advocating further investigations. Also see *S. Afr. Med. J. Journal*, Roger Wyburn-Mason, "Metronidazole in Rheumatoid Arthritis," May 1982, Vol. 61, pp. 648-649. [In personal letter to author (June 17, 1982), Paul K. Pybus, M.D. further states: "I have subsidized my treatment of this antiamoebic therapy. My intraneural treatment (developed from what was taught to me by Professor Wyburn-Mason many years ago) gives the patient immediate relief from the pain and stiffness of the disease. Metronidazole keeps them that way."

[2] Alec Hamilton died of "uncontrollable bleeding from gastric ulcers," as a result of the side-effects of corticosteroids as reported to John R. Simoons, Ph.D. via letter by A.E. Strover, M.D. of Cape Town, South Africa.

[3] According to Dr. Jack M. Blount, demographic studies ought to demonstrate a statistically significant relationship between use or exposure to copper and lessened incidence of rheumatoid diseases, as with certain primitive tribes that use copper bowls for cooking and eating, exclusively. William E. Catterall, Sc.D. and Nutritionist, in a March 23, 1983 letter to Professor Roger Wyburn-Mason, says: "I remain skeptical about your treatment of swimming pools. Concerning your evidence, many pools would be toxic to amoeba under filling conditions. I have typical water analyses around the U.S. East Coast (typically soft, acid water) with copper contents up to 5 ppm. Excess copper is likely to precipitate at typical pool pH of 7.4-7.6 and no more could dissolve. In any case, dissolution of oxide-coated copper at this pH must be nil, as suggested by non-corrosion of copper water systems at this pH. The copper algicide I mentioned is readily available in the U.S.: BioGuard® MSA Algicide (Bio-Lab, Decatur, Georgia). This contains 7% copper in the form of a soluble triethanolamine complex. The

recommended treatment is 4 oz./5000 gal., or 0.4 ppm copper added."

⁴ Bingham, Robert, M.D., **BOOK REVIEW**, *Arthritis News Today,* "The Causation of Rheumatoid Disease and Many Human Cancers, A New Concept in Medicine by Roger Wyburn-Mason, M.A., M.D.", pp. 5,6.

⁵ Professor Wyburn-Mason does not state that all of the aforementioned diseases are solely caused by the amoeba, nor that solid, unmoveable, scientific proof has been proffered in all named diseases, certain specified rheumatoid diseases certainly being an exception, in that solid scientific evidence has been presented.

⁶ *Arthritis News Today*, "What is Adequate Treatment for Rheumatoid Arthritis," Vol. 1, No. 8, May 1979, p. 7. (It should be noted that in the view of Professor Roger Wyburn-Mason, unless the amoeba is absent from the system, rheumatologist's routine more or less standard treatments involving heat and exercise may need to be re-evaluated.)

Chapter X
Is It Ethical to Deny the Sick?

Children Sick Forever —
Why haven't the various rheumatology associations and foundations and the rheumatology organizations of professional medical practitioners studied Professor Roger Wyburn-Mason's findings, now nearly a generation old?

Why does the arthritis foundation still conduct television telethons, using the names of music celebrities, *for the purpose of finding a cure for rheumatoid diseases*, when the primary cause and cure is already known?

Why are Professor Roger Wyburn-Mason's findings made known only in a book of this kind? Why isn't the whole medical profession aware of Professor Wyburn-Mason's astounding discovery?

On television yesterday I [the author] watched three lovely children limping through playground activities. Beside them was a young, handsome, learned rheumatologist, who nicely explained to us, his audience, that these children suffered from an *incurable* disease, and that their only hope lie in aspirin substitutes.

I restrained hot tears.

Suppose you *knew* for certain that these children could be cured, that the method was simple, inexpensive, eminently safe, and took but six or seven weeks? What would you do? Would you immediately pick up the telephone and try to contact that professional specialist? Would he listen if you did? What credentials do you have to make him listen? The fact *you* are cured is *not* a credential, but perhaps nothing more than a "spontaneous remission" — the modern world's name for miracle.

Or perhaps you never had the disease. Someone who was not a specialist undoubtedly diagnosed it wrongly to begin with — the proof, you understand, lies in the definition of "incurable." If the disease is incurable, then how can it possibly have been cured? And if the expert, the specialist, has pronounced it as such, i.e., incurable, then who are you to say otherwise?

The Right to Try!
Dr. Jack M. Blount records all of his telephone conversations, and one such I listened to with great dismay and shame. A specialist in rheumatology called Dr. Blount and proceeded to

lecture him with great vituperation. Was Dr. Blount *trained* in this specialty of rheumatology? If not, then what *right* did Dr. Blount have to *practice* in this field? — and so it went, until at last the caller stated, "I hope someone gets you!"

The rheumatology specialist had not heard of the brilliant medical detective work of Professor Roger Wyburn-Mason, nor had he read that the limax amoeba was the source cause of rheumatoid diseases, nor had he talked to patients who claimed to be cured, nor had he conducted laboratory examinations on them, nor had he asked for an explanation from Dr. Blount, nor had he ever tried the simple medications the knowledge of which is given away so freely — free of charge — by all participants.

Was this specialist ethical? "Is it ethical for a group of men who can offer . . . no hope whatever, to deny . . . the right to *try* a remedy of which they do not approve?"[1]

I am *not* implying that all young, learned specialists in rheumatology are so hostile, so unthinking, so unscientific, but I have been terribly amazed at the lack of response in the so-called objective field of medicine and science to Professor Roger Wyburn-Mason's nearly life-time work.

Vested Interests

We all suffer from vested interests: In the case of this brash, young, learned specialist in rheumatology, he suffered from an insufferable ego, an identification of his own personality with cookbook truisms taught him by the elite and also those who could and did decree upon him a symbol of his great value to society, his medical certificate. Can one who has studied so long, and so hard, and who is so conscientious have overlooked a genuine cure for rheumatoid diseases? In his mind, hardly! Anyone who says otherwise, therefore, must be a quack, a real danger to society!

It takes a genuinely humble, self-knowing individual to acknowledge that lessons long-learned are in error, that life is for learning, each and every day, until the very end, that we must continue to learn and unlearn.

Then there is the vested interest of State Medical Boards, each member presuming to judge peers according to standards established by state legislatures (also pressured by special interest minority groups called medical associations).

Any doctor who does not prescribe according to the current peer-group dictates of the times risks being censured by such boards, and at the very least will be embarrassingly, summarily brought before them to explain his/her peculiar behavior in treating someone in a non-standard, non-accepted, non-peer-group manner. The fact that no member of these boards has a cure to the problem is not pertinent to their hearing. In their minds the important thing is that one treats patients according to accustomed norms.

The doctor who persists in curing people with non-standard, non-accepted, non-peer-group fashion also risks legal liability suits which are not covered by medical mal-practice insurance. Apparently insurance companies also have a vested interest in covering only standard, accepted, peer-group medicine. Why should they take risks? Their job is to make money for stockholders, not to cure people. If they accept current standard, accepted, peer-group treatment procedures approved by minority groups called medical associations, then they are legally safe from law-suits, and they can maximize their profit accordingly. On the other hand, they *will* finance small pamphlets to encourage people to drive safely, to look out for household accidents, etc., such activities not requiring them to take any kind of risk at all.

Do not forget the attorney who can make a contingency fee for filing and winning a suit against a medical doctor who treats with a non-standard, non-accepted, non-peer-group procedure, and, along with him, the patient who, rather than blame God, or the devil, or his environment, or his genes, finds it more convenient to blame the one person who genuinely strives to help. It looks awfully good to a naive jury for the attorney to ask "Dr. So and So, is this procedure approved by your peers who are specialists in the field?" It is so easy to second-guess the physician, especially in the artificial environment induced by courts of law, so far removed from the problem. The fact that you have *cured* is not pertinent, apparently.

Washington bureaucrats also have their little niche to protect. More and more decision-making has descended on petty tyrants who must blindly follow rules laid down by Congressmen who also responded to special interest groups. While the U.S. Food and Drug Administration has undoubtedly saved thousands of lives by their over-protectiveness in medical applications, they have also lost thousands of lives by the same guidelines. No one counts lives lost, and no one loses jobs for it, and so ultra-conservativism is the norm when deciding to release or not to release a particular medicine for use on a particular disease. Many foreign countries have leaped ahead of the United States in medical applications, and we, the mighty and forward thinking American union of states have fallen ten to twenty years behind in certain applications.

Drug companies may apply to the U.S. Food and Drug Administration for permission to run limited tests on certain approved drugs. Treatment of arthritis by means of antiamoebic medicines should be pronounced entirely safe and easily approved — many of the indicated medicines have been in use since the sixties in the United States, for other purposes, without contra-indications. Yet this writer has read numerous letters about efforts to get various drug manufacturers off their duff, to treat arthritics with these procedures under Federal guidelines. Well, *fifteen billion dollars* returned to them annually for repetitive sales of ineffective aspirin substitutes is a larger financial stake than the total national budget of many countries. Why should drug manufacturers take the lead in cutting down their own share of the medical pie? Besides, drug manufacturers contribute a great deal of money to arthritis foundations dedicated to "finding the cure" to arthritis, and to rheumatology groups. By this means, their consciences are salved.

This author has also read numerous letters written to foundations by the esteemed participants. The foundations claim to have a vested interest in treatment and potential cure of arthritis. Letters to the foundations itemized in detail the source cause of arthritis, the nature of the amoeba involved, how to isolate it, grow it, identify it, and how to inoculate animals with it to create similar diseases as humans have, human cases cured and how they were cured, and how long were follow-ups, as well as scientific source data. These foundations generally send out a nicely printed form letter that is so insulting that they don't bear repeating in detail. In essence they say thank you for being interested in arthritis and we will file your information in our files and perhaps some day some researcher will scour through them, and he will find your note, and it will help someone, somehow!

Lastly don't forget the patient — you and I — we each have

strong-binding vested interests in maintaining our sicknesses: for sympathy, for a talking subject, for bringing about presumed companionship and ending presumed loneliness, for excuses to ourselves and others on why we cannot do things, or are not successful, for continued collection of pensions and insurance monies . . . .

Knowing all of this, what can I do to help those small, beautiful children recently viewed on television, and pronounced as forever ill, forever to be crippled, forever to be stunted. . . . ?

Definition of a Quack

According to John W. Campbell[2] "Back before Pasteur discovered germs, Semmelweis discovered a 99.9% successful method of stopping childbed fever. There was a hospital in Vienna, one half of which was run by nuns, and the other half by doctors. The incidence of childbed fever in the doctor's half of the hospital at times ran as high as 90% — [10% to 30% of the] young women who came in to have their babies died of infection. The nuns had a far better record.

"The doctors didn't observe the fact particularly; the women of Vienna were acutely aware of it, however. (The human tendency to count your hits, and forget your misses — while the women observed the misses a lot more actively.)

"Semmelweis, studying the situation, came to the conclusion that the difference was that the doctors, as part of their routine, performed autopsies on the dead women; the nuns did not. Semmelweis came to the completely false, crackpot notion that it was the odor of death on the doctors' hands that transmitted the disease. It just happened that he picked, as his deodorizer, chlorine water[3]. It did indeed deodorize the doctor's hands; also, quite unknown to Semmelweis, it was an extremely powerful antiseptic — the concentration he used would kill anything.

"At that time — about a century ago — it wasn't customary to wash the hospital sheets very often, either — until Semmelweis detected the 'odor of death' there, too. 'Wash 'em! And use chlorine water!'

"The death rate from childbed fever among Semmelweis' patients dropped from about [30% to 1.2%].

"For this, Semmelweis was thrown out of the hospital by the other doctors, and violently attacked and harassed by the medical profession of Europe.

"Why? Because of a certain emotional factor involved.

"His work — his absolutely unarguable and shocking success — said 'Doctor — healer! — *you* killed those young women. *You* killed them with your dirty hands. They didn't just 'happen to die'; *you killed them!*'

"Semmelweis was, of course, a dedicated healer; he could not endure standing idly by, so he was very busily spreading the word to laymen — telling them not to let a doctor examine a woman unless he scrubbed his hands in chlorine water.

"There's the old saying 'What you don't know won't hurt you'. With respect to objective factors, that's obviously false. With respect to emotional things, however — it's true. So long as a doctor could hold off from his own mind the realization that it truly *was* his unclean hands that did it — then he did not have the grinding agony of regret.

. . . .

". . . the modern attitude that the patient has a right to perfect security, puts the doctor under terrific pressure to refrain from *any* therapy.

"Now let's consider for a moment what's meant by a 'quack' in the medical field.

"The usual charge is that a quack is someone who uses an improper treatment, one which does not help, or actually injures the patient, while inducing the patient to pay for his mistreatment, and keeping the patient from going to a licensed doctor and getting the treatment he needs. That a quack is in the business solely to make money at the expense of suffering humanity.

"Now any time A disapproves of B emotionally, he'll attribute B's actions to some generally demeaned motivation — 'just for money' being the most common, with 'just for his own pleasure' being a runner-up.

"Let's be a bit objective about this business of what a quack does. Suppose a man, calling himself Dr. Jones, treats a patient who has a lethal disease, and uses a method he knows for a positive fact will not save the man's life. He charges fees, and sees to it that the patient doesn't go to any other therapist — just gives him some drugs that do not save him, but let him die slowly.

"That set of actions fulfills exactly what the AMA[4] accuses those awful, nasty, wicked quacks of doing.

"It is also precisely what an AMA doctor does when he treats [a certain arthritis] patient; he *knows* that the standard treatments for [arthritis] do not work, do not save lives. [Arthritis], treated by AMA methods, means [continuous pain, disfigurement and possibly] death.

"The AMA, moreover, does everything in its power to make it impossible for the victim to get treatment from any other therapist who *might* be able to do better, and most certainly couldn't be less effective.

"The patient [may], moreover, wind up broke, and his family in debt — a charge constantly leveled against those wicked quacks! — by the time he dies.

"But this is not quackary, of course.

"Why not? Because the doctors know they are doing their best, with the best of intentions — which is strictly an emotional statement.

"How about an unlicensed non-M.D. who does his best, with the best of intentions — despite the AMA's convictions that he *must* be evil — and actually does better than the AMA's best?

"Oh . . . I see. That never happens, huh. . . .?

". . . how about that unlicensed non-M.D. — that charlatan, that fraud, who'd gotten crackpot ideas from studying silk-worms and wineries, no less! — who started treating human beings for rabies? That chemist, with only half a brain, Louis Pasteur?

"Or how about that licensed M.D. charlatan, expelled from the hospital and the medical society — Semmelweis?

"Or take a few other notorious quacks like Lister — who was most violently attacked for his temerity in opening the abdomens of living patients. (Ethical doctors of the time never opened the abdomen until after the patient died.) And Ehrlich, another chemist, who invented the concept of chemotherapy.

"Every time someone outside — or even inside! — the field of medicine brings up a break-through discovery, he'll be labeled a quack. The field is too emotional.

"He'll be charged with being a fraud, a charlatan out after money, a blood-sucking leech.

. . . .

"Actually, it's pretty clear, the definition of 'quack' is 'someone I believe to be dangerous, evil, destructive and unprincipled'.

"Trouble is — the term 'quack' was — in their own place and time — violently hurled at many men we consider today among the greatest medical heroes. [Semmelweis], Jenner, Koch, Harvey, Ross, Lister, Pasteur, Ehrlich, Sister Kenny, even Roentgen, who didn't even try to practice medicine!

"One very certain thing about the field of medicine: it is not, and never will be a field of objective science. It's too deeply dominated by emotional factors."

Considering all of the above vested interests from which spring emotional factors that will blind the very best intentioned, how can one answer those who insist on clinging to old methods that are absolutely doomed to failure?

The answer, I think, is simple, indeed elegant!

Ask —

> "Have you read Professor Roger Wyburn-Mason's research work?"

> "Have you studied the many case histories that reflect 'cures' in the traditional medical sense?"

> "Have you talked to people who claim to have been cured? Have you studied their medical histories? Before and after?"

> "Have you looked into the technical, professional literature, beginning with C.A. Kofoid and O. Swezy in 1922, and terminating with Wyburn-Mason, today?"

> "Have you attempted to isolate out the thermotropic, free-living *Limax amoebae*? Grown them in the laboratory? Inoculated animals, and observed their illnesses?"

> "Have you reviewed the research and medical credentials of Professor Roger Wyburn-Mason?"

> *"Do you have any better alternative to offer?"*

State, in short, that —

> "Simple denial, quiet disclaimer, profound indifference, is no longer sufficient . That the means are at hand for your cure, for your neighbor's cure; and even though you, yourself, must also remain skeptical, you — the sick one — have an absolute right to try a remedy so safe and so economical."

I Pray That You Will Be Healed, Too!

While not in medicine, this writer does have a rather extensive life-time of readings and work in mathematics and general science, and believes himself somewhat familiar with the scientific method, bio-statistical procedures and requirements, the placebo effect and personal-emotional-involvements in one's own cures, and also in the dangers of early pronouncements regarding cures.

I have taken the time to study the authorities in the field, to read Professor Roger Wyburn-Mason's massive research report, to look at his credentials , to interview Dr. Jack M. Blount's patients, to get to know and to study Dr. Blount, to correspond with others using similar or the same techniques, and even to try the medical procedures on myself, to an almost instant and wonderfully good effect.

It is my considered opinion that Professor Roger Wyburn-Mason will one day stand with Semmelweis, Jenner, Koch, Harvey, Ross, Lister, Pasteur, Ehrlich, Sister Kenny, and Roentgen as one of the greats in medical history.

It is my considered opinion that Professor Roger Wyburn-Mason should have received the Nobel and Lasker Prizes in medicine.

It is my considered opinion, and prayer that those lovely children I recently viewed on television will be given the opportunity to be healed, as have tens of thousands since 1974!

It is my prayer that you, too, will be healed, as have I!

---

[1] Harrison, Harry, Editor, *John W. Campbell: Collected Editorials from Analog*, "Louis Pasteur, Medical Quack" (Reprint from John W. Campbell Editorial, *Analog Science Fact and Fiction*, Conde' Nast Publications, Inc., New York, NY, June 1964, p. 7), Doubleday and Co., Garden City, New York, 1966, p. 110. Permission for reprint granted by The Conde' Nast Publications, Inc. and Davis Publications, Inc..

[2] Ibid, p. 114-122

[3] There seems to be some historical conflict between references as to whether phenol (carbolic acid) or chlorine water was used. According to the *Encylopedia Americana*, Vol. 24, Grolier Inc., Danbury, CT, 1982, p. 545, Semmelweis required students to wash their hands in chlorinated lime.

[4] Although John W. Campbell has used the AMA organization as a vehicle to embellish his article, more fitting for this purpose would be use of the various arthritis foundations and the rheumatology association which, so it is said, are heavily subsidized by the drug industry, and both having to date been unwilling to look at Professor Roger Wyburn-Mason's life-time scientific work, or the results of various practicing physicians such as those reported herein.

Chapter XI
Treatment of
Osteoarthrosis, Osteoporosis
Rheumatoid Pains
and
Elements of Proper Nutrition

The "Aging" Disease

Somewhere in man's long history he accepted the idea that there are diseases "caused by aging." Such diseases, of course, can not be halted. One gets old, and one "ages" and one degenerates slowly but quite surely, until at last other infectious diseases brings us to our maker; or we break our bones and become invalided and dependent upon others for a mere pittance of unhappy survival.

Among these "aging" diseases *that everyone knows* is that of osteoarthritis, a disease of the "aging" that affects approximately 90 per cent of the population by the age of 40. Among the many symptoms, degenerative joint diseases is the most common cause of chronic disability.[1]

When the author wrote the first edition of this book to report on the wonderful news that rheumatoid disease can and is being cured by a simple, low-cost medicine, there was no intent to include osteoarthritis. *Everyone knew* that osteoarthritis is *completely* unrelated to rheumatoid disease: rheumatoid disease displays systemic infectious factors (although its agent was unknown until Professor Roger Wyburn-Mason's research), whereas osteoarthritis was considered as simply a consequence of being human — and living long enough. One lived through time, and one *aged*, and one got degenerative bone and joint diseases. The "wear and tear" disease, it was called, although no authority ever bothered to check the mechanical engineering of human joints with mechanical and materials engineers, who would have informed that the bones and joints should be good for 150 years or more, based on simply the mechanics.

So much for "wear and tear —."

We victims of rheumatoid disease often also have mingled with our systemic rheumatoid symptoms, osteoarthritic symptoms, as well as weakening of the bones, called osteoporosis, where the ratio of bone cell replacement to bone cell destruction has decreased, until the bones become brittle[2].

In one person, all three symptoms present themselves — or one of the symptoms may dominate over others.

Some 30 years ago, in the fifties, Dr. Paul K. Pybus worked and studied under Professor Roger Wyburn-Mason who, you may keep in mind, was a specialist in several fields, including that of diseases of the nervous system.

Roger Wyburn-Mason developed a theory of the causation of osteoarthritis which apparently was layed to rest until Dr. Paul K. Pybus had a need for it in treating members of his South African retirement community, many of whom suffered from classical osteoarthritis, and many of whom had a mingling of rheumatoid disease and osteoarthritis.

Casting back in his mind to the teachings of his earlier mentor, he came upon Roger's theory, which was that *whatever the source, osteoarthritis was a disease caused by inflammation of certain nerves, at certain key junctions,* which caused joints to stay compressed, and thereby to deny cartilage nutrients required for health.

Many who have rheumatoid disease also have osteoarthritis, and since many with osteoarthritis also display the Herxheimer effect when given anti-ameobics — even in the absence of rheumatoid disease factors — it appears as though some osteoarthritis is caused by the *Limax amoeba.* That is, with a certain affinity for nervous tissue, the *Limax amoeba* apparently also invades these key nervous tissue junction points, creating inflammation, and thereby bringing about some osteoarthritis.

Some osteoarthritis responds to treatment of anti-viral medicines, and therefore some osteo must be caused by viruses.

Some osteoarthritis responds to treatment of appropriate doses of vitamins A, D, and Calcium, and therefore some osteo must be caused by improper nutrition, or utilization of nutrition (mal-absorption often accompanies effects of rheumatoid disease.)

Surely, some osteoarthritis must be caused by bacterial agents and mechanical shock or damage, also.

In any event, in addition to a metabolic imbalance, most all osteoarthritis seems to have a common underlying cause: that the nervous tissue at certain key junctions is disturbed, becomes inflammed, sends signals to affected joints, and creates a condition where the joint cartilage cannot any longer receive proper blood supply, and therefore the cartilage begins to die — thus, "osteoarthritis," *disease of the aging.*

Dr. Paul K. Pybus[3] developed a simple technique and used it on aging members of the retirement community under his care. His results were phenomenal. *To this date he's had great success — far, far greater than traditional treatment — in treating thousands of patients! Many reportedly now conduct handball and other hitherto forbidden exercises.*

After rheumatoid disease has been vanquished — the disease process — there is left-over damage to tissues and joints that create great pain. Killing the limax amoeba, remember, does not straighten out joints, nor does it eliminate pain resulting from nerve damage done by genetic susceptibility to the amoeba.

The pain left over from rheumatoid disease is virtually identical to that found in osteoarthritis, and may be treated exactly the same way with great success.

Gus J. Prosch, Jr., M.D. was the first American to learn Dr. Paul K. Pybus's technique and to apply it to patients, including the author, with success equal to that of Pybus. Now many American Physicians have equal success. Dr. I.H.J. Bourne, General Practitioner, Hornchurch, Essex, reported *independent* development of identically the same technique as that developed by Dr. Pybus[4].

What follows is a second protocol from *The Rheumatoid Disease Foundation*, relating to rheumatoid disease, osteoarthrosis and osteoporosis.

It is included in this book because of the many letters and phone calls relating to osteoarthritis and the pain of rheumatoid arthritis, and is proferred here primarily for your family doctor. Gus J. Prosch, Jr., M.D. chaired the committee that wrote this portion of our treatment protocol.

The Roger Wyburn-Mason
&
Jack M. Blount Foundation
for Eradication of Rheumatoid Disease
Rt. 4, Box 137, § Franklin, TN 37064 § *(615) 646-1030*
"The Rheumatoid Disease Foundation"
A non-profit, charitable, tax-exempt organization

The Rheumatoid Disease Foundation,
**through its Board Member physicians, has established standards of practice
in the treatment of rheumatoid disease
and hereby supplements with the following protocol
when treating osteoarthrosis disease.**

Primary Osteoarthritic Disease &
Secondary Arthritis from Rheumatoid Diseases

This work and the various intraneural injection techniques were pioneered by Dr. Paul K. Pybus of Pietermaritzburg, South Africa, as a development of what was taught him by the late Professor Roger Wyburn-Mason.

He has been successfully using these techniques for over seven years for the treatment of any type of inflamed joint, and tender neuritic areas that are located near the joints. These areas are physiological disturbances in nerves. These neuromata, as they are called, affect C type nerve fibres which are responsible for the severe deep pains so often experienced in arthritis. These C type nerve fibres are 0.5-0.2mm in diameter, and have a slow conduction rate of 0.5-2.0 m/sec. When irritated, these axons generate impulses both in the normal or prodromic, and reverse or antidromic directions. Prodromic impulses, producing the sensation of slow pain, relay in the cells of the spinal cord, reflexly causing spasm or stiffness of the musculature near the joint. The antidromic impulses dilate the blood vessels in the region of the peripheral origin of the nerve fibres, causing an increase in blood supply and swelling that occurs in the distal end of the sensory nerve, and effusion into the joint.

Many of these unmyelinated C fibres travel to the various joints of the body and are very susceptible to damage which produces:
1. Pain and tenderness at the site of injury to reflexly produce:
2. Spasm of the muscles around the joint causing stiffness to produce:
3. Compression of the joint to produce:
4. Arrest of circulation of the joint fluid in the cartilage to produce:
5. Death of the cartilage cells to produce:
6. Creaking or crepitus, inflammation, swelling, heat, redness and loss of function.

It must be remembered that cartilage has no capillaries or blood vessels in it at all. Circulation in the cartilage takes place by means of joint fluid. This joint fluid is alternately sucked in or squeezed out by the cartilage, which acts like a sponge, expressing from the cartilage the nutrient synovial fluid as pressure is applied to it, and re-absorbing it again when pressure is taken off. If the muscles are continually in spasm, fluid is constantly driven out of the cartilage and so prevents circulation of the nutrients from

100

reaching the vital areas. This results in cell death, some deformity in the erosion of the joint surface, and osteoarthrosis. It is the stiffness of the muscle spasm which is responsible for the destruction and not necessarily the pain.

Therefore, in summary, it will be noted that around inflammed joints will be observed certain areas of tenderness.

These trigger points or neuromata correlate closely with the sites of various superficial peripheral nerves, and at these points the nerves are liable to damage. Around these damaged nerves develop areas of electrical disturbance resulting in a barrage of both antidromic and prodromic impulses arising at these points. Prodromic impulses are relayed to the dorsal horn of the spinal cord to produce a reflex spasm of the muscles around the joints, causing compression of the joint cartilage, interfering with the cartilage's nutrition and resulting in arthrosis. The antidromic impulses are conducted peripherally to the plain nerve ending where they result in the release of histamine like substances and vaso-dilatation and swelling, producing arthritis. (See Schematic Drawing I, page 102, of these nerve fibers affecting joints, suggested by Dr. Paul K. Pybus.)

If these inflammed nerves which give off so many abnormal impulses can be suppressed, there will be an immediate cessation of the pain as well as of the spasm and stiffness and a reduction in the creaking of the joints and crepitus. Blocking these impulses with local anaesthetic results in just this, namely the abolition of these impulses and the immediate cessation of their effects with restoration to normality. This, of course, only lasts as long as the local anaesthetic action persists. By adding a very small amount of depot steroid, *which remains primarily at the inflammed area*, the inflammation is finally relieved and the arthrosis and arthritis stopped, and usually permanently so.

The following table refers to schematic drawings II, III, and IV, pages 105, 106, and 107, respectively:

Technique of Intraneural Injections

The following intraneural recommendations are suggested by the foundation.

1. Palpate with firm pressure by using fingers or a blunt instrument, (e.g. pencil eraser) over any expected points of tenderness, and if tender, mark with a skin pencil. **Only the tender points are marked for injection.**

2. Infiltrate a bleb of local anaesthetic intradermally at each site of tenderness. A Dermajet® power gun is nearly painless and saves time. [Mada-jet®: Mada Medical Products, Inc., 60 Commerce Rd., Carlstadt, N.J. 07072 as per John Baron, D.O.]

3. To 10 ml 1/2% local anaesthetic add 0.25% ml (5mg) triamcinolone hexacetonide (Aristospan® or Lederspan®). This fluid should now have a milky appearance. Not more than a total of 30 ml of the mixture should be injected at any one session into the various marked points. Should the patient complain of dizziness the procedure should not be continued further, but the remaining points should be treated at a later date.

4. Introduce the needle through the local bleb and probe gently towards the expected situation of the nerve, until the patient feels pain. It is essential to watch the patient's face at this time.

5. As the patient experiences pain, (with a change of facial expression), start to inject the mixture 1-4cc.

6. The patient will experience acute pain for about 2-3 seconds.

7. All tender sites are injected in this manner, and the patient is told the numbness will last 4-5 hours and then return to normal. Explain that some bruising will occur and the sites will be sore for a day or two, but the arthritis pain will no longer be there. If the nerves are injected properly, relief of the pain usually lasts from 4 months to 5 years or longer, but the overall average is about one year.

8. The patient is seen after one week and any points still tender are injected again. This can be repeated at weekly intervals until all pain is gone. The patient is then seen at three-monthly intervals and any recurrences dealt with as necessary.

Schematic Drawing I

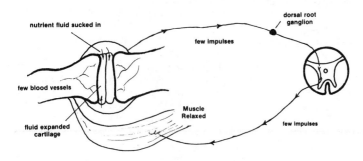

**NORMAL POSITION
OR WHEN COMPRESSION IS TAKEN OFF**

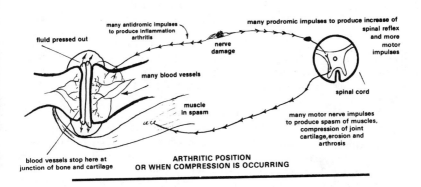

**ARTHRITIC POSITION
OR WHEN COMPRESSION IS OCCURRING**

Probable cause of pain in osteoarthrosis according to Professor Roger Wyburn-Mason and Dr. Paul K. Pybus, who also developed a successful remedy. These two pictures occur alternately when the patient is walking. However, when the nerve has been inflamed, as in the above picture, the cartilage stays pressed and nutrients do not provide for the cartilage, and it is destroyed.

Injection Points for Intraneural Injections

Injection	Acupuncture	Nerve Root	Name of Nerve	Location of Tender and Injection Points and Details of Possible Variations
#1	BL-9	C-2	Greater occipital	Lateral aspect of upper margin of external occipital protuberance about 1 inch from midline
#2	GB-11	C-2	Lesser occipital	On posterior aspect of mastoid process of temporal bone about 1-3/4 inch lateral to #1
#3	BL-10	C-3	Third occipital	Approximately 2 inches inferior to #1 and 3/4 inch lateral to midline
#4	TH-23	Trigeminal	Zygomatico-temporal	Two centimeters above zygomatic arch at the lateral tip of the eyebrow
#5	BL-2	Trigeminal	Supraorbital	At the medial end of the eyebrow
#6	SI-17	C-2,3	Great auricular	At point where external jugular vein crosses anterior border of sternomastoid
#7	HT-1	C-5,6	Axillary (lower branch) (Circumflex humeral)	In mid-axilla on medial aspect of axillary artery
#8	Not Known	C-5,6	Axillary (upper branch) (Circumflex humeral)	Just dorsal to anterior axillary fold or crease
#9	TH-13	C-5,6	Lateral cutaneous of arm (Circumflex)	On posterior surface of arm approximately 1-2 inches lateral to posterior axillary fold
#10	SI-9	C-5,6	Axillary bifurcation	One thumbsbreath superior to posterior axillary fold
#11	SI-10	Brachial Plexus	Suprascapular	Passing through suprascapular notch sending filaments to all joints of shoulder
#12	CO-15	C-3,4	Supraclavicular (Posterior branch)	Posterior-lateral and inferior to acromion where depression is formed with arm raised
#13	TH-15	C-3,4	Supraclavicular (Anterior branch)	Posterior over trapezius muscle 2-3 inches lateral to midline at level of C-4
#14	BL-41	C-6,7,8	Thoracodorsal	Four fingerbreadths (of patients) or 3-1/2 inches lateral to inferior end of spinous process T2
#15	SI-12	C-5,6	Superior subscapular	In middle of supraspinatus fossa
#16	LU-5	C-5,6,7	Lateral cutaneous of forearm	At cubital fossa on the radial aspect of biceps tendon
#17	SI-8	C-8, T-1	Medial cutaneous of forearm	Anterior to medial epicondyle of humerus with elbow flexed. (May be found as the nerve emerges through the deep fascia in front of medial epicondyle
#18	HT-3	C-5, 6, 7, 8, T-1	Median	F-3. Never used.
#19	LU-8, 9	C-5, 6, 7, 8, T-1	Anterior inter-osseous	Never used.
#20	TH-4	C-5, 6, 7, 8, T-1	Posterior inter-osseous	On the dorsum of the wrist in the depression of the skin crease proximal to the 3rd and 4th
#21	CO-4	C-5, 6, 7, 8, T-1	Radial terminal branches	On dorsum of hand in anatomical snuff box
#22	SP-20	T-2, 3	Lateral pectoral nerve	Six inches lateral to mid-sternal line at a line even with the 2nd intercostal space
	SP-21	T-6	Lateral cutaneous	In the mid-axillary line in the 6th intercostal space
#23	KI-27	T-1	Anterior cutaneous	One and 3/4 inches lateral to mid-sternal line in the 1st intercostal space
	KI-26	T-2	Anterior cutaneous	One and 3/4 inches lateral to mid-sternal line in the 2nd intercostal space
	KI-25	T-3	Anterior cutaneous	One and 3/4 inches lateral to mid-sternal line in the 3rd intercostal space
	KI-24	T-4	Anterior cutaneous	One and 3/4 inches lateral to mid-sternal line in the 4th intercostal space
	KI-23	T-5	Anterior cutaneous	One and 3/4 inches lateral to mid-sternal line in the 5th intercostal space
	KI-22	T-6	Anterior cutaneous	One and 3/4 inches lateral to mid-sternal line in the 6th intercostal space. . .etc.

Injection Points for Intraneural Injections

Injection	Acupuncture	Nerve Root	Name of Nerve	Location of Tender and Injection Points and Details of Possible Variations
#24	BL-27	S-1	Posterior rami S-1	One to 1-1/2 inches lateral to 1st sacral vertebra, superior to sacroiliac joint
#25	BL-28	S-2	Posterior rami S-2	One to two inches lateral to 2nd sacral vertebra, superior to sacroiliac joint
#26	BL-29	S-3	Posterior rami S-3	One to two inches lateral to 3rd sacral vertebra, level with anterior superior crest of ilium
	BL-30	S-4	Posterior rami S-4	One to two inches lateral to sacral hiatus
	BL-35	S-5	Posterior rami S-5	One centimeter lateral to the mid-line of spine, level with the superior border of the coccyx
#27	BL-37	S-1, 2, 3	Posterior femoral	Trigger points can be anywhere in a 2 inch band running down the mid-posterior thigh from the gluteal region to the back of the knee
#28	GB-27, 28	L-2, 3	Lateral femoral cutaneous	Anterior and about one inch inferior to the anterior superior spine of the ilium
#29	LI-11	L-2, 3, 4	Accessory obturator	Approximately one inch inferior to medial end of Poupart's ligament
#30A B	None known	L-2, 3, 4	Obturator	A. Anterior area of greater trochanter; insert needle at X and penetrate to trochanter.
			Nerve to rectus femoris	B. Superior area of greater trochanter; insert needle at X and penetrate to trochanter.
C			Nerve to quadratus femoris	C. Posterior area of greater trochanter; insert needle at X and penetrate to trochanter.
#31	GB-30	L-2, 3, 4	Joint capsule femoris (Hip)	Two thirds of distance from midline on a line joining the greater trochanter with sacral hiatus
#32	ST-34	L-2, 3, 4	Intermediate femoral cutaneous	Two to three thumbsbreadths superior to the patella
#33	SP-10	L-2, 3, 4	Medial femoral cutaneous	Two thumbsbreadths superior to the medial border of the patella with the knee flexed
#34	SP-11	L-2, 3, 4	Saphenous in femoral canal	Approximately 6 inches superior to #33 on the medial aspect of Sartorius muscle and lateral to the femoral artery
#35	GB-31, 32	L-2, 3	Lateral femoral cutaneous	On the lateral aspect of the thigh approximately 4 to 6 inches proximal to the superior border of the patella
#36	SP-9	L-2, 3, 4	Saphenous	At attachment of median longitudinal ligament 1-2 centimeters inferior to medial condyle of tibia about 1 inch medial to patella; this point often relieves ankle pain
#37	?	L-2, 3, 4	Saphenous	At origin of infrapatellar branch of the nerve
#38	?	L-2, 3, 4	Saphenous	Immediately below the patella; there may be two or three points located here
#39	?	L-2, 3, 4	Saphenous	At the apex of the curve in the nerve as it enters the subcutaneous tissues
#40	ST-36	L-4, 5	Musculocutaneous (Peroneal)	Approximately 3 inches inferior to tibial tuberosity and one finger lateral to crest of tibia in the tibialis anterior muscle
#41	SP-6	L-2, 3, 4	Saphenous for foot	At the junction of the mid and lower 1/3 of the shaft of the tibia approximately 4 inches superior to the apex of the medial malleolus and slightly medial to tibial crest
#42	LI-4	L-2, 3, 4	Saphenous for foot	At the lower 1/4 of the tibial shaft two thumbs superior to the medial malleolus and lying just medial to the tibial crest
#43	ST-41	L-4, 5 / S-1, 2	Anterior tibial (Deep perineal)	On dorsum of foot in the center of the inferior extensor retinaculum and between the tendons of the extensor hallucis longus and extensor digitorium longus
#44	BL-59, 60	L-4, 5 / S-1, 2, 3	Sural	In the depression anterior to the Achilles tendon and posterior to the lateral malleolus. Also three inches superior to this point

Nerve Sites for Intraneural Injection

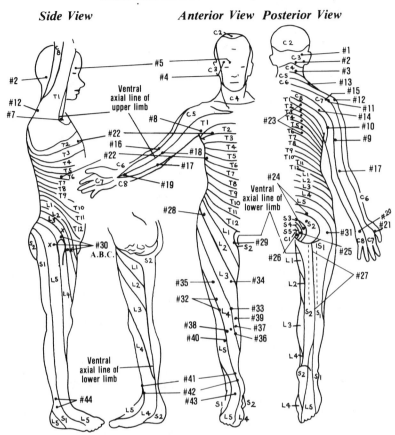

Side View   *Anterior View*   *Posterior View*

Schematic Drawing II

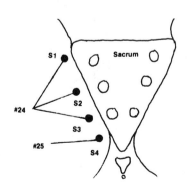

Points for Sciatica

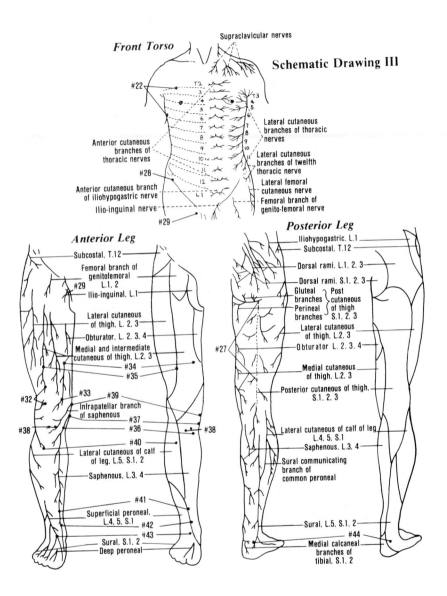

Front Torso

Supraclavicular nerves

Schematic Drawing III

#22

Anterior cutaneous branches of thoracic nerves

#28

Anterior cutaneous branch of iliohypogastric nerve

Ilio-inguinal nerve

#29

Lateral cutaneous branches of thoracic nerves

Lateral cutaneous branches of twelfth thoracic nerve

Lateral femoral cutaneous nerve

Femoral branch of genito-femoral nerve

Anterior Leg

Subcostal, T.12

Femoral branch of genitofemoral L.1, 2

#29
Ilio-inguinal, L.1

Lateral cutaneous of thigh, L. 2, 3

Obturator, L. 2, 3, 4

Medial and intermediate cutaneous of thigh, L.2, 3

#34
#35

#32
#33 #39

Infrapatellar branch of saphenous

#37
#38 #36

#40

Lateral cutaneous of calf of leg, L.5, S.1, 2

Saphenous, L.3, 4

#41

Superficial peroneal, L.4, 5, S.1
#42
#43

Sural, S.1, 2
Deep peroneal

#38

Posterior Leg

Iliohypogastric, L.1
Subcostal, T.12

Dorsal rami, L.1, 2, 3

Dorsal rami, S.1, 2, 3

Gluteal branches   Post
Perineal   cutaneous
branches   of thigh S.1, 2, 3

Lateral cutaneous of thigh, L.2, 3

Obturator L. 2, 3, 4

#27

Medial cutaneous of thigh, L.2, 3

Posterior cutaneous of thigh, S.1, 2, 3

Lateral cutaneous of calf of leg, L.4, 5, S.1

Saphenous, L.3, 4

Sural communicating branch of common peroneal

Sural, L.5, S.1, 2

#44

Medial calcaneal branches of tibial, S.1, 2

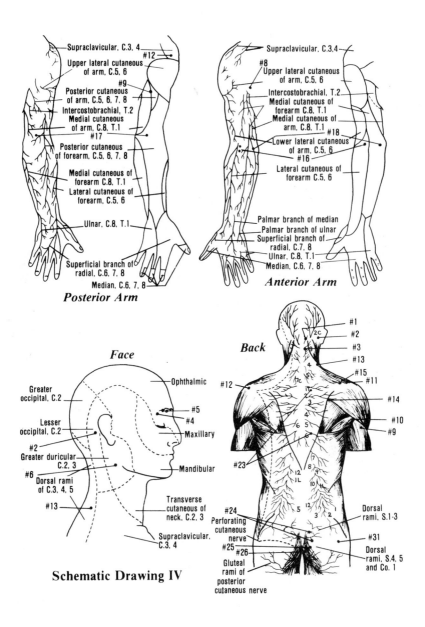

Posterior Arm

Supraclavicular, C.3, 4
#12
Upper lateral cutaneous of arm, C.5, 6
#9
Posterior cutaneous of arm, C.5, 6, 7, 8
Intercostobrachial, T.2
Medial cutaneous of arm, C.8, T.1
#17
Posterior cutaneous of forearm, C.5, 6, 7, 8
Medial cutaneous of forearm, C.8, T.1
Lateral cutaneous of forearm, C.5, 6
Ulnar, C.8, T.1
Superficial branch of radial, C.6, 7, 8
Median, C.6, 7, 8

Anterior Arm

Supraclavicular, C.3,4
#8
Upper lateral cutaneous of arm, C.5, 6
Intercostobrachial, T.2
Medial cutaneous of forearm C.8, T.1
Medial cutaneous of arm, C.8, T.1
#18
Lower lateral cutaneous of arm, C.5, 6
#16
Lateral cutaneous of forearm C.5, 6
Palmar branch of median
Palmar branch of ulnar
Superficial branch of radial, C.7, 8
Ulnar, C.8, T.1
Median, C.6, 7, 8

Face

Greater occipital, C.2
Lesser occipital, C.2
#2
Greater auricular C.2, 3
#6
Dorsal rami of C.3, 4, 5
#13
Ophthalmic
#5
#4
Maxillary
Mandibular
Transverse cutaneous of neck, C.2, 3
Supraclavicular, C.3, 4

Back

#1
2c
#2
#3
#13
#15
#11
#12
#14
#10
#9
#23
#24
Perforating cutaneous nerve
#25 #26
Gluteal rami of posterior cutaneous nerve
Dorsal rami, S.1-3
#31
Dorsal rami, S.4, 5 and Co. 1

Schematic Drawing IV

107

Recommendations, Rationale and Research

The majority of physicians working with *The Rheumatoid Disease Foundation* are realizing the importance of good nutrition, adequate and proper diet with necessary vitamin and mineral supplementation. With the increasing number of patients being treated by these physicians daily, a few obvious facts are becoming clearer. Those of greater importance are the following:

1. Most all arthritic patients' body fluids are more acid than they should be.
2. Most all arthritic patients show numerous signs and symptoms of a deficiency in free or ionic calcium in the body.
3. Most arthritic patients drink 2% butterfat milk, eat margarine instead of butter and demonstrate a lack of Vitamin D and A along with other nutrients.
4. The diet of arthritic patients does play an important part in controlling the severity of their symptoms.
5. Vitamin and mineral supplementation does shorten recovery time and by strengthening the immune system, these patients become less susceptible to reinfection by the amoebae as well as other infections.

As opinions and conclusions tend to vary widely at the present time among most physicians concerning the use of diet, vitamin and mineral supplementation, and strengthening the immune response system, *The Rheumatoid Disease Foundation* makes no recommendation to any physicians concerning these important factors. These decisions are left to the discretion of the attending physician. However, to those physicians who are sincerely interested in these important factors and especially as to the trend in thinking of most physicians working with *The Rheumatoid Disease Foundation* who seriously consider these factors, a short summary of diagnostic signs and symptoms and our rationale concerning diet, vitamin and mineral supplementation and strengthening of the immune system will be presented.

Credit for much of the following information should be given to Carl Reich[5], M.D. of Calgary, Alberta, Canada who has intensely studied much of the presented information for the past twenty years. Dr. Reich has noticed a strongly positive relationship between the various forms of arthritis and poor or inadequate nutrition. Numerous other physicians have observed similar findings along with a multitude of arthritic patients. One of our physicians has undertaken a continuing in-depth study of this subject, resulting in three primary observations:

1. Many patients who are blood-related to arthritic persons do not develop arthritis especially when different dietary habits are followed.
2. Oftentimes arthritic patients exhibit slight to significant improvement when self-administered home and folk remedies are taken, as alfalfa tablets, bone meal tablets, cod liver oil capsules, vinegar with honey, peanut oil, bee venom and cherries.
3. Some patients are more susceptible to becoming reinfected with the amoebae than others, once the germs have been destroyed in their bodies by antiamoebic drugs.

The same physician initiated a program to accomplish the following three proposals listed below. Space does not permit a detailed explanation of the techniques and methods of study involved, and so only conclusions are presented.

Studies Performed

1. To determine any previously overlooked physical signs and symptoms exhibited primarily by arthritic patients.
2. To determine and correct any poor or inadequate eating habits along with any vitamin and mineral deficiencies present by using an in-depth and detailed past history questionnaire.

108

3. To determine a successful method to strengthen the arthritic patient's immune system in an effort to prevent any reinfection by the amoebae along with any simple and easy-to-follow techniques that will rid the patients drinking water of any pathogenic amoebae.

Tentative Results of These Studies

1. There are present with arthritic patients certain physical signs and symptoms which has been found to be much more prevalent than in normal persons not afflicted with arthritis. Of course one must understand that not all arthritic patients exhibit every sign or symptom listed below but some are seen in nearly every arthritic (rheumatoid and osteo) patient in one form or another:

   a. Longitudinal ridges in fingernails with an increase in opaqueness of the nails.
   b. Mild to moderate tenderness with strong palpation of the soleus and trapezius muscles.
   c. Generalized slight increase in deep tendon reflexes.
   d. Generalized irritability of skeletal muscles to percussion.
   e. Acid saliva on the average should be about pH 7. Arthritic patient's saliva usually ranges from 4.5 to 6.5 as determined by using Hydrion® paper which is manufactured by Micro Essential Laboratories of Brooklyn, N.Y.
   f. Slight to severe coating on the tongue.

2. An in-depth past history questionnaire which includes a past nutritional evaluation should be completed on arthritic patients. Most arthritics consume a diet that is strongly acid-forming in nature; and it is felt that these patients should be educated as to the proper foods they should eat along with foods they should avoid. It has been found that arthritic (rheumatoid and osteo) patients respond to treatment more rapidly and successfully when they follow the diet recommended below. The diet also helps prevent reinfection by the amoebae when followed.

Diet, Vitamins and Minerals

One of our leading physicians says:

"In my practice, I have noticed that most arthritics avoid whole milk and butter and instead drink skim or low-fat milk and eat margarine. Their clinical symptoms and physical examination signs usually demonstrate strong evidence of a deficiency of "free" calcium in their system as well as a lack of vitamins A and D. Blood calcium studies are misleading since they measure the free calcium along with other forms as all the calcium bound to proteins. Whereas normal body fluids are nearly always slightly alkaline, as opposed to acid, I constantly find those patients with rheumatoid disease have body fluids that are more acid in nature than normal. This is partly due to a deficiency in free (ionic) calcium, which in itself is very alkaline in nature, but the primary cause of this acid-alkaline reversal can be found in the diet and nutritional habits of those with rheumatoid disease. Most cellular mechanisms of the body and particularly those involving the use of ionized (free) minerals such as the secretory (all glands) processes, nerve function processes and muscle contraction, etc., proceed best in a mildly alkaline body state. For this reason, a diet consisting of high alkaline forming foods should be consumed, combined with the avoidance of acid forming foods. Acid forming foods are those which are high in one or more of three elements: phosphorus, sulfur and chlorine. Alkaline forming foods are those which are high in one or more of four other elements: potassium, calcium, magnesium, sodium. The following diet has proven to be effective in preventing and treating those with rheumatoid diseases, but also seems to strengthen and fortify an individual's immune system and body defenses, especially when combined with adequate vitamin and mineral supplements.

"The diet used to treat and prevent development of rheumatoid diseases should definitely *avoid*, as much as possible, the following foods: All processed and most canned

109

foods should be avoided along with caffeine, sugar in all its forms, as well as the simple carbohydrate foods that quickly upon digestion turn into sugar as white flour foods, crackers, many cereals, macaroni (pasta foods), white rice and corn products. Ideally nicotine and alcohol should be avoided, along with any sweets, candy, soft drinks, pastries or desserts. The "nightshade plants" (foods containing solanines) such as white potatoes, tomatoes, egg plant and garden peppers should be avoided. Also avoid chocolates since they contain oxalates which interfere with calcium absorption. Most fruits are alkaline forming (contrary to public opinion) with the exception of cranberries, plums and prunes, which of course should be avoided.

"Concerning vitamin and mineral supplementation the most important point to consider here is to correct the free calcium deficiency present in most arthritics. This requires much larger amounts of Vitamin A and D in their natural form than what is usually recommended by the 'recommended daily allowances' tables. The synthetic Vitamin A and D-2 preparations on the market simply do not work. Synthetic Vitamin D-2 does increase the calcium absorption from the small intestine but seems to be totally inadequate in regulating the use of the calcium and especially calcium excretion by the kidneys. The only preparation I have found that is adequate is the natural D-3 which is found in fish liver oils. Therefore I recommend plain cod liver oil as the ideal which seems to be even better than cod liver oil capsules. It is easily taken when mixed with some orange juice and stirred rapidly. The preparation recommended is plain Norwegian cod liver oil liquid which contains 10,000 units of Vitamin A and 1000 units of Vitamin D per teaspoon. I recommend that patients take two teaspoons on arising each morning and two teaspoons at bedtime. This preparation can be found in most health food stores and should be taken for at least four months then the dosage should be cut in half. I explain to the patients to not fear any Vitamin A or D toxicity with this dosage as it is less than 1/3 the toxicity level that has been reported in the literature. If the patient absolutely cannot take the liquid they can usually find capsules at a health food store which will provide approximately 40,000 units of Vitamin A and 400 units of D. I also explain that *exposure to the sunshine of at least 20 minutes weekly will activate the Vitamin D.*

"Concerning calcium preparations, I have found that none of the available inorganic calcium preparations are effective. I discovered that organic bone meal tablets (3-4 per day) work better than other calcium preparations but I continued to have reservations. Recently, I located a calcium preparation that seems to work ideally. This compound is Calcium Orotate which is the naturally occuring calcium in plants. Miller Pharmacals of Chicago or Lanpar Corporation in Dallas, Texas carries this compound and I prescribe 500 mg. Calcium Orotate (50 mg. elemental calcium) three times daily with meals for two months, then 500 mg. twice daily. This calcium preparation also seems to enhance the ability of the body to use and metabolize other forms of calcium ingested. I also prescribe 500 mg. Magnesium Orotate once daily to balance the calcium-magnesium ratio. The above calcium preparation is also excellent for osteoporosis and it greatly strengthens the bone and cartilage structures in the body."

"As a rule, most protein foods tend to be acid forming since they contain phosphorus and sulphur. Animal sources of protein — lean meat (beef, lamb, veal) poultry, fish and eggs — are definitely in this category. With the exception of shrimp, most sea food is extremely acid forming. These foods *must not* be avoided however in the diet, as they provide the building blocks for all body functions and processes. Therefore one of these proteins should be eaten with each meal. Pork meats should be limited however. Just try not to eat an entire meal consisting of protein foods, but balance these foods with alkaline forming foods. Ideally your breakfast should always consist of some high protein foods, balanced with whole milk, fruit juices, etc. Also remember to cook protein foods at low temperatures, as enzymes and trace minerals are reduced when foods are heated above 120 degrees F.

"Avoid processed and hydrogenated, or "hardened" oils and fats. Most margarines, peanut butters, restaurant prepared french fries and potato or corn chips are prepared with hardened oils. Sweet cream butter is best and use "non hydrogenated" vegetable oils (like "Pam®") for home cooking. Also watch those high calorie salad dressings. Most fats and fatty foods (butter, oils, sausages, bacon, etc.) are neutral in their acid-alkaline content but they greatly contribute to excessive weight gain which severely complicates arthritis. Therefore, it would be wise to limit all oily, greasy, fried, fatty foods, if you tend to be overweight.

"Most all vegetables (except corn) are highly alkaline in nature and should be emphasized in your eating program. Salad vegetables are excellent and should be eaten daily. All other vegetables are very good and when "wok" cooked or stir-fried in "non-hydrogenated" vegetable oil they are even better for you. Fresh vegetable juices (not canned) are nearly perfect and should be part of your diet. It is important to prepare and serve as many foods in their raw and natural state as possible. All fruits and fruit juices (excepting cranberries, plums and prunes) are very good alkaline forming foods and should be eaten daily. Most nuts (with the exception of peanuts, pecans and walnuts) are alkaline forming and are good to "munch" on. Whole milk is one of the best alkaline forming foods due to it's high calcium content. Raw certified whole milk is much preferable if you can find it and I would class it as the #1 choice of foods for arthritis patients. You should not drink skim milk or low fat milk in preference to whole milk. At least two glasses of whole milk should be taken each day and use butter instead of margarine. Plain yogurt is an excellent alkalinizing food and not only is easy to digest but tastes great when mixed with fresh fruit. Certain dried fruits such as raisins, dates, dried figs and apricots are also good and make excellent munching foods. This diet will change your system to be more alkaline as it should be.

[It is also reported that the steroid, Decadurabolin® (nandrolone decanoate by Organon) injected intra-muscularly, 100 mg. once each month for six months, also reverses the progress of osteoporosis — Editor.]

"Concerning other vitamins for arthritic patients, I recommend as an ideal supplement program the following: .

1. Vitamin B Complex — two to three "Stress" B vitamins daily in divided doses.
2. Vitamin C — two to three grams daily in divided doses.
3. Zinc Orotate — 500 mg., one to two tablets daily.
4. Selenium 250 micrograms daily as yeast selenium.
5. B-Carotene — 25,000 units daily.
6. Vitamin E — 400 units daily.

"The above vitamin and mineral supplementations will not only help the patient's arthritis by stimulating the immune response system but will play an important role in counteracting the ageing process as well as acting as a deterrent to some forms of cancer since many of these preparations act as free radical and peroxide scavengers in the body. With painful hands and feet I recommend in addition 100 mg. Vitamin B6 twice daily. This is also helpful for carpel tunnel syndrome. With neuralgia I suggest 500 mg. niacinamide twice daily.

"In treating rheumatoid disease patients who have recently been taking any cortisone preparations, gold injections or penicillamine, the physicians working with *The Rheumatoid Disease Foundation* have discovered that these patients respond more slowly and less effectively with anti-amoebic medications. Professor Roger Wyburn-Mason believed that these medications produce some form of shield or coating around the amoebae which prevents the anti-amoebic drug from getting to the amoebae.

"In trying to prevent reinfection of the amoebae and realizing that drinking water is a primary source of reinfection along with the fact that copper kills the amoebae effectively, the writer recommends to patients that they should either boil their drinking water 10-15

111

minutes before drinking or to place one half pound of clean "non-insulated" copper wire in each of two gallons of water which is allowed to stand at least 8 hours before drinking.

The Rheumatoid Disease Foundation recommended treatment for rheumatoid arthritis was previously presented in Chapter IV. Dr. Prosch's observations (which coincide with some *Foundation* members' observations) on osteoarthritis follow:

1. It has been observed that the majority of osteoarthritic patients are infected to some degree with the amoebae. For this reason, all osteoarthritis patients are first given a "therapeutic trial" of anti-ameobic medication usually in the form of metronidazole and allopurinol as suggested under the recommended techniques of treating rheumatoid disease.

2. Location and injection of tender points of the nerves affecting the involved joints as shown under the prior table and schematics in this section under intraneural injections.

3. Prescribe amantadine hydrochloride (Symmetrel®) 100 mg. three times daily for 2-3 months or until symptoms disappear. Along with this, colchicine 0.6 mg. should be given once daily for 6 days of each week for 2-3 months or until well. These two together (without other treatment) have proven effective in about 55% of patients, according to Dr. Archimedes A. Concon.

4. Follow the recommended diet suggestions to "alkalinize" the body.

5. Follow the recommended vitamin and mineral supplementations mentioned previously with special emphasis on the proper dosage of cod liver oil and calcium, magnesium and zinc orotates.

This protocol is subject to revisions (additions, deletions, changes) as Board Members complete relevant research.

Perry A. Chapdelaine, Sr.
Executive Director/Secretary
As of March 1984

[1] *Fifteenth Edition of the Cecil Textbook of Medicine, Vol. I*, W.B. Saunders Co., Philadelphia 1979, p. 202.

[2] Deca-durabolin®, used in South Africa and Europe, seems to turn osteoporsis around. See *The Rheumatoid Disease Foundation* protocol, "Diets, Vitamins, and Minerals."

[3] See *The Control of Pain in Arthritis of the Knee*, Paul Notrik, *The Rheumatoid Disease Foundation*, Rt. 4, Box 137, Franklin, TN, $4.50 plus $1.00 postage and handling, 1984.

[4] See "Treatment of Backache with Local Injections," 222, 708-711; "Treatment of Painful Conditions of the Abdominal Wall With Local Injections," 224, 921-925; "A Controlled Trial to Compare the Effects of Local Injection of Corticosteroid and Lignocaine into Painful Lesions of the Back"; "Treatment of the Painful Knee With Local Injections" all with *The Pracitioner*; "Local Injection Therapy," *The Physician*, 185-188, 1984.

[5] According to Carl J. Reich, M.D.: "In essence I feel that calcium is intimately related with energy release mechanisms of the cell and deficiency of it enhances these processes to cause "burn out" of cell function, whether it be of muscle cell, nerve cell, connective cell, etc.

"Likewise I feel that calcium deficiency causes the autonomic nervous system to excite certain adaptive units, present in the lung, intestine, or skeleton to function in a different direction that may be compensatory for the encroaching calcium deficiency state.

"These combined influences of calcium ion deficiency of course, may be heightened by any toxin which will depreciate the effectiveness of ionic calcium.

"Therefore a calcium deficient patient may be asymptomatically adapting to the calcium deficiency by some autonomically excited process of lung, intestine and skeleton and in such instances this asymptomatic adaptive process may be broken down to pathological maladaptive disease by an infection which may aggravate the deficiency state.

"Most importantly, vitamin A which is the natural accompaniment of vitamin D and calcium in milk products, and vitamin A which accompanies vitamin D in fish oils, may be a natural anti-yeast or protozoal protective device, the deficiency of which will predispose the individual to infection with these agents. Because of the co-existence of these nutrient factors in milk products and fish oils etc., the person who becomes infected for reason of vitamin A deficiency, naturally pays the penalty of experiencing the calcium disrupting effect of the toxin which the infection excretes.

" . . . Possibly the most important aspect . . . [the] symptoms and signs due to the direct effect of deficiency on the individual, may constitute a warning that the person's deficiency is of a level that is exciting physiological adaption. I now also interpret these symptoms and signs as a warning that the individual also is susceptible to infection, which infection may depreciate the asymptomatic adaptive device to pathological expression in acute fashion, whereas otherwise, if infection did not occur, the breakdown of this function to induce disease might not have occurred for years or decades later, or possibly not at all."

[6] *Patient Nutrition Handbook*, Nettie F. Strauss, National [now Desert] Arthritis Medical Clinic, 13-630 Mountain View Road, Desert Hot Springs, CA 92240; *1981 Arthritis Program*, Robert Bingham, M.D., same address.

[7] ANAVIT-F3, Chemical Consultants International, Inc., P.O. Box 88041, Honolulu, Hawaii, 96815.

Chapter XII
The Past and the Future

The BCF Syndrome

For people like you and I, the future is again glistening. Not only do we perceive the living of useful, happy pain-free lives, but through forthcoming research of the tax-exempt, non-profit *The Rheumatoid Disease Foundation we perceive discovery and development of new techniques and medicines that will prevent tissue and joint destruction before it begins. Before the tuberculosis bacillus was discovered, physicians had a hundred different names for what seemed to be a hundred different diseases. Once the tubercle bacillus was identified and isolated, it became apparent to all that what had come in a hundred different guises was in reality but one germ that affected a hundred different body tissues.*

Thus it is also for Professor Roger Wyburn-Mason's discovery of the Limax amoeba — a hundred different symptoms disguised by discriminating medical nomenclature now is found to have the same basis, and therefore the same cure.

Since the first edition of this book the author has repeatedly been asked: "Why don't the authorities — medical organizations, drug manufacturers, Arthritis Foundation, U.S. Government, et. al. — look into Professor Roger Wyburn-Mason's findings, and do something about all this? After all, they are in the business of helping the sick."

I thought that Chapter X, "Is It Ethical to Deny the Sick?" with its inclusion of a description of vested interests, sufficient to answer the question in advance. It appears that something stronger is required.

There is a sickness among us which I've titled the *BCF Syndrome*:

> This disease is characterized by a group of mental disorders affecting thinking, mood and behavior. There is an altered concept of reality, and in some cases delusions and hallucinations. Mood changes include inappropriate emotional responses and loss of empathy. Withdrawn, regressive, and bizarre behavior may be noted. Whenever reality is addressed; i.e., whenever the

115

person's attention is forcibly directed toward the real-world, delusions of persecution may drive the individual to attack with unwarranted venom. Such attacks often take the form of Authoritarian statements of denunciation to the press, radio, and TV, the primary purpose of which is to restore the denouncer to a semblance of inner security in an inner world where all things are nicely predictable, thus also nicely controlled, and no thing is perceived as a threat.

I am writing, of course, of the dreaded BUMBLEBEES CAN'T FLY SYNDROME.

The BUMBLEBEES CAN'T FLY SYNDROME was named during the first part of this century in the 1920's or 1930's (I believe) by some unknown scientist who, when shown certain mathematical equations clearly demonstrating that Bumblebees Can't Fly, said, "But what of the one that has just flown to your shoulder?" He was summarily drummed from the Scientific Academy and thereafter attacked in the news media with great venom, many claiming that he was a fraud, a charlatan, not a true scientist at all: and at least one great organization, *The Foundation for the Preservation of the Mammoth Elephant*, proceeded forthwith to send out a stupendous number of requests for research funds to find the cure on why Bumblebees Can't Fly, at the same time warning all recipients not to listen to any quacks who claimed otherwise.

While the disease — BCF SYNDROME — was named but recently, the symptoms were observed several hundred years ago, the most memorable occasion being when august French scientists at a famous museum threw out a valuable collection of meteorites, patiently collected over several hundred years, because "everyone knew that rocks can't come from the sky."

Of course, I'm being facetious!

But consider the same thought posed in a more restrained manner: Arthur Koestler in his *The Sleepwalkers*[1], says:

".... the inertia of the human mind and its resistance to innovation are most clearly demonstrated not, as one might expect, by the ignorant mass — which is easily swayed once its imagination is caught — but by professionals with a vested interest in tradition and in the monopoly of learning. Innovation is a twofold threat to academic mediocrities; it endangers their oracular

116

authority, and it evokes the deeper fear that their whole laboriously constructed intellectual edifice may collapse."

Consider, for example, the Arthritis Foundation: It ought've done something with Professor Roger Wyburn-Mason's research the moment it was published, in 1964, but they did not. In the author's opinion, and to the author's personal knowledge, the Arthritis Foundation has impeded any attempts to spread the word, or to bring about proper scientific investigation of Professor Wyburn-Mason's work — and it still begs for money "for research to find the cure for arthritis!"

Most of the established Foundations use a code word that, among those not in the know, sounds erudite and conservative and proper; but in fact, to those who are in the know — the medical and scientific establishment — means "don't touch" *we* haven't approved. That code word is simply *not proved* or "an unproven remedy." The term "unproven remedy" is fostered on the public as being equivalent to quackary — this despite the fact that 80-90% of AMA-approved medical practices are also unproven, according to the *U.S. Office of Technology Assessment*, publication (1978), "Assessing the Efficacy and Safety of Medical Technology." Try calling the Arthritis Foundation and ask why they are not using and/or propagating the Roger Wyburn-Mason treatment which has been said to be scientifically proved over six years ago. The answer you will most probably receive from any of its many branches will be simply "not proved." This code word means "not invented here," "not approved by our FNR (friendly neighborhood rheumatologists) who run our organization," "boycott this treatment, because it's not part of *our* establishment," and so on. They will never once tell you that they are themselves investigating the claims — for they are not —, or that they've furnished funds for running "requisite" double-blind studies — for they have not —, or that they have looked into the claims, either through Professor Roger Wyburn-Mason's research, or through other physician's cures and remissions — for they have not.

They will never tell you of the eminent research background, in many medical fields, of Professor Roger Wyburn-Mason, but rather seek to cast doubt on this wonderful person through innuendo and false statements taken out of context. And when they speak of Dr. Jack M. Blount, of course, they will use two

117

modes: (1) On the record, this is an "unproven" remedy (the code word), and they will make fun of his heart-rending story as told herein in Chapter II. (2) Off the record, Dr. Blount is a [you fill in the blank].

The Arthritis Foundation has over many years used its IRS tax-exempt base and its privilege of free radio and TV time to *condition* people into believing that their foundation is the sole authority on arthritis, that everyone else who has insight, knowledge, data, is a fraud and charlatan, that one should check with *them* before making any move whatsoever. They admittedly can do nothing for you, except teach you how to live with your pain and suffering and continuing and increasing disfigurement, but since they've set themselves up as being *The Authority*, they have the gall to also judge for you where to go for treatment — and they will protect your pocketbook from charlatans and con artists while steering you to your FNR (friendly neighborhood rheumatologist), who will take your money without any cure, instead.

The Arthritis Foundation has no greater legal basis for existing than does any other association of individuals; nor are they any greater authority than they can produce workable results — which is apparently none!

As to the FNR (friendly neighborhood rheumatologist) he or she is a physician who has specialized in rheumatology. Consciously or unconsciously professional rheumatologists know that if Professor Roger Wyburn-Mason is correct, and that rheumatoid diseases can be easily and swiftly cured with a small amount of medicine (and they can), then *any general practitioner can cure the disease, and rheumatology as a speciality is doomed!* Some, I'm sure, have a severe mental conflict when they are told that all the procedures they use, for treatment and for alleviation of symptoms, are wrong! After all *they* are the experts. They've a university degree to show for it, haven't they? The fact that they cannot get results is ignored by their own suffering from the BUMBLEBEES CAN'T FLY SYNDROME

As to how the American petro-chemical industry, the American health systems, and some foundations, control virtually all practice of medicine for profit (as opposed to the chief aim of getting people well) I have only to refer the reader to a series of *Penthouse* articles wherein thorough investigative and objective reporting shreds the mysterious veil of direct and indirect control over the American publics' right to health[2].

And any serious student of these matters would do well to review problems encountered by The Dreyfus Medical Foundation[3], wherein Jack Dreyfus, — who had access to Presidents, top Federal bureaucrats and the Army Surgeon General — was unable to effect a needed minor change in the *Physicians Desk Reference*[4]. One famous German physician describes Americans as "Stupid," because we conduct all the basic medical research, and then bury it. All the Europeans need do is read our journals, and apply findings and lo!, they are ahead of us in medical applications by twenty years!

It is not the author alone, and other now-cured rheumatoid victims who have reached the point of disgust on how our health and welfare is controlled by others with vested and narrow-viewed interests. The People's Medical Society[TM][5] has recently been chartered with the stated goals of giving each of us more control over our own medical care and to reduce health-care costs. Robert Rodale, says, "The medical confrontation is not just coming — it's here[6]."

The Rheumatoid Disease Foundation

The Roger Wyburn-Mason and Jack M. Blount Foundation for the Eradication of Rheumatoid Disease, IRS tax-exempt, non-profit, is dedicated to curing you, and everyone else who suffers from rheumatoid diseases: (1) stop disease progress, (2) repair damage, (3) maintain health.

Professor Roger Wyburn-Mason spent many agonizing years suffering through skeptical rebuffs, when all anyone had to do was look at his profferred research. Jack M. Blount, Jr. M.D. likewise has charged ahead despite much ridicule and persecution to bring his knowledge to those who, like himself, also suffered.

Every member of *The Rheumatoid Disease Foundation* has sacrificed more or less in some manner to bring this valuable information to those who suffer needlessly.

With welcome assistance from many others, *The Rheumatoid Disease Foundation* is now sending out letters asking for research funds to bring Roger Wyburn-Mason's findings to fruition. There are many research, development, and application needs that can be satisfied through your donation — big or small — and these are:

1. First and foremost is the use of funds to conduct "double-blind" studies. We must demonstrate to the American medical

and scientific establishment the correctness of Professor Roger Wyburn-Mason's treatment. In making "double-blind" studies, patients are divided into two groups, one to receive the medicines that are thought to cure or bring relief, and the other group that receives a known neutral ingredient, called a placebo. "Double-blind" studies means that neither the patient nor the physician is aware of which patient receives the anti-amoebic and which the placebo (inert ingredient without any medicinal value). In some parts of Europe it is both unethical and illegal to perform double-blind studies when an agent is known to effect relief of pain and suffering. In the United States it is necessary to convince those who set the standards (medical establishment) of what shall constitute proper medicinal treatment, although neither the miraculous sulfa drugs nor penicillin went through such costly and extravagant studies. Perhaps double-blind studies can be effective in showing which of several anti-inflammatory substances, that treat symptoms only, is most effective, but of what use when the cause and cure are known? *The Rheumatoid Disease Foundation* has acquired funds through generous donors, and is currently running double-blind studies with clotrimazole at Bowman Gray School of Medicine, Winston-Salem, NC, Department of Rheumatology under Robert Turner, M.D. These scientific studies will take 12 months, but as studies begin, it will be quickly shown that double-blind studies cannot be done, because each infected patient who receives antiamoebics will have the Herxheimer effect, and the administering physician will at once know which patient is receiving the antiamoebic and which is not, thus destroying the "double-blind" aspect. However, *The Foundation* must go through this expensive charade for the sake of getting information into the present hard-headed medical establishment.

There are another $2,000,000 worth of studies of similar nature waiting to be funded.
2. There must be developed a better test to determine genetic susceptibility to the *Limax amoeba* in advance of tissue destruction, and awaiting the Jarisch-Herxheimer effect (after taking antiamoebics) for initial verification. Right now it's like saying, "Yup! That guy over there who's almost dead *did*

have the disease." Until now the state of medical art has precluded such definitive tests — most expensive presently used laboratory tests and x-rays are non-definitive — but whole new fields of bio-genetic engineering are unfolding which give promise to solve this problem neatly[7].

During 1985, with the help of generous donors, this *Foundation* will fund one to three university centers to duplicate Roger Wyburn-Mason's initial work in isolating the limax amoeba. When this step is accomplished, we will then be able to fund monoclonal antibody studies that will provide the physician with a specific test to determine which amoeba must be killed by which antiamoebic. No more guessing or shotgun approach!

3. Now that we know how insidiously dangerous is the *Limax amoeba* we should have a catalog of all 300 or more species, with their characteristics, so that basic and developmental research can be performed to safeguard people; such research would include knowledge on how they affect changes in tissues, their capacity to adapt to changing environments, including different antiamoebics, their relationship to diets, including vitamins and minerals — and we must communicate to people on the proper procedure of treating the symptoms of rheumatoid disease. For example, for many years rheumatologists have told victims to exercise, and to use massage and warmth. It turns out that this standard advice has been causing the organism that causes rheumatoid disease to spread faster. Money must be spent to de-condition people, so that they will know the truth.

We must have definitive tests that can discriminate between allergies, yeast infections, bacterial, viral, and amoebic.

5. *The Rheumatoid Disease Foundation* will republish Professor Roger Wyburn-Mason's masterly publication, *The Causation of Rheumatoid Disease and Many Human Cancers*[8] and his *Addenda*[9]. These must be made more widely available so that all physicians and scientists can study in detail the massive amount of work Wyburn-Mason placed into them over a lifetime, and thereby convince themselves that merit lies therein.

6. Other rheumatoid diseases that have not, until now, been recognized as related to the rheumatoid condition need more

studies and therefore also need funded. Many have been named in chapter VII, but it would be well to cover here two important ones: cancer and multiple sclerosis.

In Wyburn-Mason's *Addenda*[10] is stated: "Certain human lesions are well recognized as premalignant and, if their cause could be elucidated and removed, the possibility of finding the aetiology and of prevention of some forms of cancer arises." Wyburn-Mason briefly reviews the statistical studies, and their implications, and it becomes easy to visualize that perhaps as much as 20% of cancer is now set up by the *Limax amoeba* by establishing a changed environment around individual cells, which, when the cells adapt because of the changed environment, become "precancerous," among which are the following: Exocrine glands (salivary and lacrimal glands, cystic mastitis, chronic lymphocytic pancreatitis, liver), Endocrine glands (lymphocytic or Hashimoto's thyroiditis, adrenal, parathyroid, thymus, ovary), Mucosa of the respiratory or gastrointestinal tract, Colon, Lungs, Gallbladder, Bone Marrow, Bones, Lymph Nodes, Macroglobulinaemia, etc. Wyburn-Mason further states, "In order to prevent certain malignant changes it would seem that the premalignant lesions described above must be prevented. This can be accomplished in some cases by the administration of antiamoebic substances to all subjects at regular intervals as every person becomes reinfected with amoebae in the course of his life and these may be pathogenic or the subject sensitive to them. In this way [the various syndromes] can be prevented."

Multiple sclerosis, the last disease researched by Wyburn-Mason before his death, also seems to be an invasion of the central nervous system by *Limax amoebae*. However, those antiamoebics now routinely used to cure other rheumatoid diseases are dangerous for victims of multiple sclerosis to use, because during the course of killing the amoebae, there is a plaqueing over of nervous tissue, causing the disease to progress faster. Obviously, now that the cause of multiple sclerosis is known, research funds for assessing anti-amoebics which do not at the same time create a worsening condition would be very well spent. Since the cause of multiple scelorsis is known, the disease can now be prevented by assuring that those who are susceptible to the *Limax amoeba* receive antiamoebics before the disease progresses into the nervous structure; and perhaps the cure of multiple sclerosis is just around the horizon, as has already been experienced by other rheumatoid disease victims. As of this writing, one of our cooperating physicians *may* have the answer for MS! Perhaps by the next book's edition we will be privileged to publish that answer.

7. Since the *Limax amoeba* is resistant to chlorine, the treatment of public water systems must be reevaluated, and public hygiene programs must be instituted for preventing reinfection through swimming pools, drinking water, mishandling of sewage, and so forth.

8. Perhaps one or more clinics for the indigent can be established across the nation and the world in time. Cost is no longer a large factor in treating rheumatoid victims.

9. Hundreds of thousands of antiamoebics need to be screened to learn which are the most effective. Those given in this book, Chapter V, represent chiefly the results of discoveries by Prof. Roger Wyburn-Mason, Jack M. Blount, M.D., and Robert Bingham, M.D., none of whom have been in the business of searching and screening. Think of what can be found — and the good that will be forthcoming — when funds are at last available to search out the most effective, lowest cost antiamoebics!

The above are only my suggestions. *The Rheumatoid Disease Foundation* Board Members will make a determination of priorities as donations become available, and you can be quite sure that any further suggestions, whether or not accompanied by a donation to *The Foundation*, will be seriously considered.

Donations

If you are concerned for yourself, your children and their children, and other loved ones, and if you want to help in this magnificent effort, your donation may be made to *The Rheumatoid Disease Foundation*, P.O. Box 17405, Washington, D.C. 20041. Your gift will be tax-deductible, and will represent a first effort to lick a scourge that has been with man since his beginnings, and must, therefore, be an act of mercy heard by many sufferers and also by *He* who demands love and mercy for us all —.

[1] Koestler, Arthur, *The Sleepwalkers*, McMillan Co., New York, New York, 1959.

[2] Some of the articles are: "The Great Cancer Fraud", Gary Null and Robert Houston, *Penthouse*, 909 3rd Ave., New York, New York 10022, September 1979; "The Suppression of Cancer Cures", Gary Null, *ibid*, October 1979; "Alternative Cancer Therapies", Gary Null with Anne Pitrone, *ibid*, November 1979; "Suppression of New Cancer Therapies: Dr. Joseph Gold and Hydrazine Sulfate", Gary Null with Anne Pitrone, *Ibid*, January 1980; "The Politics of Cancer, Part 5 — Suppression of New Cancer Therapies: Dr. Lawrence Burton", Gary Null and Leonard Steinman, *ibid*, July 1980; "The Politics of Cancer, Part 6 — Suppression of Alternative Cancer Therapies: Dr. Josef Issels", Gary Null and Leonard Steinman with Kalev Pehme, *ibid* August 1980; "The Politics of Cancer, Part 7 — Laetrile — The Drug That Never Was", David Rorvik, *ibid*, January 1981; "The Politics of Cancer, Part 8 — The National Cancer Institute", Allan Sonnenschein, *ibid*, July 1981; "The Politics of Cancer, Part 9 — The Cancer Insurance Scam", Robert Sherrill, *ibid*, January 1982; "The Politics of Cancer, Part 10 — Warning: The American Cancer Society May be Hazardous to Your Health", Allan Sonnenschein, *ibid* May 1982; "The Politics of Cancer — The Promise of Hydrazine Sulfate" Ralph W. Moss, *ibid*, January 1983.

[3] *A Remarkable Medicine Has Been Overlooked*, Jack Dreyfus, Pocket Books, 1230 Avenue of the Americas, New York, New York 10020.

[4] *Physicians Desk Reference*, Medical Economics Co., Inc., Oradell, New Jersey 1983.

[5] People's Medical Society™, "Charter Invitation", Trieste Kennedy, 33 East Minor Street, Emmaus, Pennsylvania 18049.

[6] "Our New Alliance For Health," Robert Rodale [with the magazine editor], *Prevention*, 33 East Minor Street, Emmaus, Pennsylvania 18049, May 1983.

[7] "Antibodies for Sale," Julie Ann Miller, *Science News*, Vol. 123, No. 19, May 7, 1983, pp. 296-298, 302

[8] *The Causation of Rheumatoid Disease and Many Human Cancers — A New Concept in Medicine*, Roger Wyburn-Mason, Iji Publishing Co., Tokyo, Japan, 1978.

[9] *The Causation of Rheumatoid Disease and Many Human Cancers— A New Concept in Medicine, A Précis and Addenda, including the Nature of Multiple Sclerosis,*, Roger Wyburn-Mason, AC Projects, Inc., Rt. 4, Franklin, TN 37064, 1983

[10] *Ibid*, pp. 15-17.

Chapter XIII

Dr. Jack M. Blount's Suspended Sentence

The Board Hearing

In 1983 Dr. Jack M. Blount received a suspended sentence of two years from the State Board of Medical Licensure of Jackson Mississippi. Dr. Blount's "crime" was, as follows:

> Following a hearing before the Board of Medical Licensure on May 19, 1983, and July 21, 1983, Dr. Blount was found guilty of unprofessional conduct, which included, but was not limited to, making or wilfully causing to be made many flamboyant claims concerning his professional excellence and he was judged guilty of dishonorable or unethical conduct likely to deceive, defraud or harm the public . . . the Board suspended Dr. Blount's Mississippi medical license No. 2466 for a period of two (2) years. However, the period of suspension was stayed upon Dr. Blount's compliance with certain conditions:
>
> Dr. Blount shall cease issuing papers extolling the particular virtues of the expected results of his treatment for arthritis.
>
> Dr. Blount shall not prescribe by mail or in person to a patient unless he has conformed to the traditional ethical medical methods, including but not limited to, the taking of a medical history and performing a physical examination and suitable laboratory procedures.
>
> Dr. Blount shall post conspicuously in his office a statement that the treatment he uses for arthritis is *experimental* and that there is no guarantee of any cure.
>
> Dr. Blount shall verbally inform each patient he treats for arthritis that the treatment he uses for arthritis is *experimental* and that there is no guarantee of any cure.
>
> Dr. Blount shall personally reappear before the board after a period of one (1) year has elapsed.
>
> If Dr. Blount fails to comply with any of the conditions it will result in the immediate lifting of his license to practice medicine in Mississippi.
>
> Dated July 25, 1983 — Mississippi State Board of Medical Licensure

As with most Board Hearings and court cases, the public seldom views behind scenes, they seldom sense or know the prejudicial power vectors that thrust a man like Dr. Jack M. Blount before a set of supposed peers for judgment. Fortunately the author has personal and private knowledge that can shed some light on what took place, and by means of this book you, the reader, can know something of those forces in our society that fight to keep us from getting well:

Prior to Blount's hearing of May 19, 1983, this writer got word from an independent source that the Arthritis Foundation had taken action to "get" Dr. Jack M. Blount, and next to go after another of *The Rheumatoid Disease Foundation* Board Members.

As reported in Chapter II and Chapter III of this book, Dr. Jack Blount was miraculously cured of arthritis himself, and he passed

125

his good news on to this writer and to thousands of others. In perhaps 127 patients (including this writer), Dr. Jack Blount, gave prescriptions away *free of charge*. When the prescriptions were used properly, sick people got well, or at least much, much better. It was perhaps unethical, by current medical practices, to give prescriptions away to those who had not been seen in his office, but how much more unethical would it have been for Dr. Blount to deny desperately ill people the same relief he had achieved?

His Hippocratic oath as a physician required that he service suffering mankind — but his license as a Mississippi doctor required him to deny those same suffering people.

What would you do, knowing that you could easily lift your brother's burden by means of three scraps of paper: three prescriptions sent free of charge and with tons of love —?

During the hearing, Dr. Blount was repeatedly accused of making flamboyant claims. You, the reader, can judge Dr. Blount's judges: Read again Chapter II of this book, and ask yourself if Dr. Blount was making flamboyant claims. This chapter is a reprint of a speech Dr. Blount gave to a local business organization in Philadelphia, Mississippi immediately on recovering from death's tolling, and it was later used to tell people about his swift recovery and what he'd discovered, using Professor Roger Wyburn-Mason's theory and recommendations. According to the prosecutor (and the Board), Dr. Blount must not use the words "miracle" and "cure". For him to use these words is the making of flamboyant claims. In retrospect it seems quite obvious that had Dr. Blount told each and every patient: "Look! God is not involved in my sudden, new and wonderful knowledge, only science," and "There is no miracle, I cannot cure you or bring you relief," (a lie) then Dr. Blount, like all Friendly Neighborhood Rheumatologists, would not have been accused of the making of flamboyant claims.

There is an obvious constitutional question of whether or not any Board has the right to control another American's speech, writing, or religious convictions. I was taught that we were all guaranteed the right of freedom of worship, belief, and the right to freedom of speech and writing. Regardless of your conviction or mine, to permit Dr. Blount's freedom of speech and religious convictions to be restricted, even in part, also decreases our own personal freedoms, and that of our loved ones.

It is the author's opinion, and hopefully the readers, that the Mississippi Board had no right to delve into Dr. Blount's religious

126

expression or right to express his opinions — to patients or anyone else.

Dr. Jack M. Blount was brought before the Board by entrapment. Someone (probably the Arthritis Foundation) put the bug in one of the Mississippi investigative agencies, and told them to entrap Dr. Blount.

Of all the witnesses brought before the Board, only one was not a member or agent of the investigative agency set out to trap Dr. Blount. Each member but the one told essentially the same story to the Board: They were called on to lie to Dr. Blount about their desperate sickness and need for help, and they lied about their inability to come to his office, and they lied about their inability to pay. Thinking each to be a legitimate brother in sickness, Dr. Blount sent the same prescriptions that cured this writer, each free of charge.

The prescriptions were not used by these liars, of course, and were offered as part of the case against Dr. Blount.

The sole witness that was not (apparently) a direct agent of the Board, became one through intense fears placed in her by jealous rheumatologists or the Arthritis Foundation or the investigative agency or some combination of the three.

In her testimony on the stands she said exactly the words that the Board's prosecutor had coached her to say, in the writer's opinion. But her words and emotional mannerisms told another story, that of a sickly woman who had been terrified by falsehoods, and she was stimulated to hostility and now wanted to get even.

She had been told by someone unknown that Dr. Blount's prescriptions were dangerous, and that she must not take them. She was obviously still ill with severe rheumatoid disease, and I introduced myself to her as a writer, and asked if I might talk to her for a short time. I had hopes of convincing her that she would be well if she tried those simple remedies.

The opposing attorney got wind of my plans and immediately ushered the lady away from me, and out of the hearing room — gone forevermore. This action, more than any other single action at the "trial", gave lie to the supposed ethics and purposes of the investigative agencies that performed the entrapment proccesses.

My final observation in the hearing is that the prosecutor at all times held two things on trial: (1) Dr. Jack M. Blount's giving away of free prescriptions, and (2) Professor Roger Wyburn-Mason's "unacceptable" theory of cause and treatment of rheumatoid diseases.

While an equal amount of hearing time was spent on both portions, in all fairness to the Mississippi Board, they did not charge Dr. Blount with the requirement that he stop treating people according to the new methods and techniques, nor did they pronounce that the treatment and cure were fallacious.

They were wise to bear restraint —!

Additional General References

A medical doctor has so few courses in protozoology that it is unlikely the average physician will know much about amoebic infections. The following references, for the most part, are tendered for those who would like to gain a better knowledge of amoebae characteristics, and some of its slow-growing research and clinical history.

Abd-Rabbo, Hassan. "Dehydroemetine in Chronic Leukaemia." *The Lancet*, 1161-1162, May 21, 1966,.

_____. "Chemotherapy of Neoplasia (Cancer) with Dehydroemetine." *J. Trop. Med. Hyg.*, Vol. 72, 287-290, 1969.

_____. "Is Flagyl Dangerous?" *The Medical Letter on Drugs and Therapeutics*. Vol. 17, No. 13 (Issue 429) 53, June 20, 1975.

Abd-Rabbo, H.; H. Abaza, G. Hillal, M. Moghazy, L. Asser. "Nitro-imidazole in Rheumatoid Arthritis," *Am. J. Trop. Med. Hyg.* 75, 64-66, 1972.

Adam, Katherine M.G. "A Comparative Study of Hartmannellid Amoebae." *J. Protozool.* 11(3), 430-435, 1964.

Ahn, Tae I., Kwang W. Jeon. "Structural and Biochemical Characteristics of the Plasmalemma and Vacuole Membranes in Amoebae." *Exp. Cell Res.* 137, 253-268, 1982.

Albanese, A., Anthony, A. Herbert Edelson, Edward J. Lorenze Jr., Maurice L. Woodhull, Evelyn H. Wein. "Problems of Bone Health in Elderly." *New York State Journal of Medicine.*, 326-336, Feb. 1975.

Anderson, Hamilton. "The Use of Fumagillina in Amoebiasis." *Annals New York Academy Sciences*, 1118-1124, 1952.

Anderson, Kevin, Adele Jamieson. "Primary Amoebic Meningoencephalitis." *The Lancet*. 902-903, April 22, 1972.

Anonymous. "Amoebic Meningo-encephalitis." *The Medical Journal of Australia*, Vol. 1, 1036-1038, May 17, 1969.

_____. "Legionella and Amoebae." *The Lancet*. March 28, 703-704, 1981.

_____. "Pathogenic Free-living Amoebae." *The Lancet*. Dec. 3, 1165-1166, 1977,.

Anderson, K. & Jamieson, A. "Primary Amoebic Meningoencephalitis." *The Lancet.*, 902-903, April 22, 1972.

Apley, J., S.K.R. Clarke, A.P.C.H. Roome, S.A. Sandry, G. Saygi, B. Silk, D.C. Warhurst. "Primary Amoebic Meningoencephalitis in Britain." *British Medical Journal*. 596-599, March 7, 1970.

Arehart-Treichel, Joan. "Boning Up On Osteoporosis." *Science News*. Vol. 124, 140-141, Aug. 27, 1983.

Armstrong, J. & Pereira, M. "Identification of 'Ryan Virus' as an Amoeba of the Genus *Hartmannella*." *British Medical Journal*. Jan. 28, 212-214, 1967,.

Balamuth, William. "Action of Antibiotics Against Intestinal Amoebae *In Vitro*." *Annals New York Academy of Sciences*, Vol. 55, 1093-1103, 1952.

_____. "Comparative Action of Selected Amebicidal Agents and Antibiotics Against Several Species of Human Intestinal Amebae." *The Am. J. Trop. Med. and Hyg.*, Vol. 2, 191-205, 1953.

Beaver, Jung, & Cupp. "Pathogenic Free-Living Amebae: *Naegleria* and *Acanthamoeba*." *Clinical Parasitology*. Lea & Febiger, Philadelphia, 9th Edition, 135-148, 1984.

Bhaduri, K.P. "Endamoeba Histolytica in Leukorrhea and Salpingitis." *Am. J. Obst. & Gyn.* V. 74, 434, 1957.

Bhagwandeen, S., R.F. Carter, K.G. Naik, D. Levitt. "A Case of Hartmannellid Amebic Meningoencephalitis in Zambia." *Am. Jour. Clin. Path*. Vol. 63, 483-492, April 1975.

Bhagwandeen, S.B., R.F. Carter, K.G. Naik, D. Levitt. "A Case of Hartmannellid Amebic Meningoencephalitis in Zambia." *Am. J. Clin. Path*. Vol. 63, 483-492, April 1975.

Bisno, Alan L. "Acute Rheumatic Fever: Current Concepts and Controversies." *Current Clinical Topics in Infectious Diseases*. (Ed. Jack S. Remington, Morton N. Swartz) McGraw Hill Inc., Vol. 5, 316-341, 1984.

Blake, David R., Nicolas D. Hall, Paul A. Bacon, Barry Halliweli, John M.C. Gutteridge. "The Importance of Iron in Rheumatoid Disease." *The Lancet*. 1142-1144, Nov. 21, 1981.

Bonnin, N. & Kay, H. "Dysenteric Arthritis: Case Reports and Comments." *The Medical Journal of Australia*. Vol. 2, 380-382, 1943.

Borochovutz, Dennis, F.F. Paul, A. Julio Martinez, Gary T. Patterson. "Osteomyelitis of a Bone Graft of the Mandible with *Acanthamoeba castellanii* Infection." *Human Pathology*, Vol. 12, No. 6, 573-576, June 1981.

Bourne, I.H.J. "Local Injection Therapy," *The Physician,*" 185-188, Nov. 1984.

_____. "Treatment of Chronic Back Pain." *The Practitioner*. Vol. 228, 333-338, March 1984.

_____. "The Treatment of Pain With Local Injections." *The Practitioner*. Vol. 227, 1877-1883, December 1983.

_____. "The Treatment of Painful Conditions of the Abdominal Wall With Local Injections." *The Practitioner*. Special Report, Vol. ?, Pages 3, Date Unknown.

Bos, H. J. "A Case of *Acanthamoeba* Keratitis in The Netherlands." *Trans. Roy. Soc. Trop. Med. Hyg*. Vol. 75, No. 1, 86-91, 1981.

Bossche, H. Van, G. Willemsens, W. Cools, W.F.J. Lauwers, L. Le Jeune. "Biochemical Effects of Miconazole on Fungi. II. Inhibition of Ergosterol Biosynthesis in *Candida Albicans*. *Chem. Biol. Interactions*. 21, 59-78, 1978.

Boyle, A.J., R.E. Mosher, D.S. McCann. "Some *In Vivo* Effects of Chelation — I Rheumatoid Arthritis." *J. Chron. Dis*. Vol. 16, 325-328, 1963.

Brewerton, E. Albert. "Rheumatology." *HLA and Disease*. Ed. Dausset, Jean, Arne Svejgaard. Williams & Wilkins Co., Baltimore. 94-107, 1977.

Butt, Cecil. "Primary Amebic Meningoencephalitis." *The New England Journal of Medicine*, Vol. 274, No. 26, 1473-1476, June 30, 1966.

Butt, C., Baro, C. & Knorr, R. "Naegleria (sp) Identified in Amebic Encephalitis." *The Am. J. of Clinical Path*. Vol. 50, No. 5, 568-574, 1968.

Callicott, Jr., Joseph H., E. Clifford Nelson, Muriel M. Jones, Joao G. Santos, John P. Utz, Richard J. Duma, Joseph V. Morrison, Jr. "Meningoencephalitis Due to Pathogenic Free-Living Amoebae." *JAMA*. Vol. 206, No. 3, 579-582, Oct. 14, 1968.

Cantwell, Alan R. Jr. "Histologic Forms Resembling 'Large Bodies' in Scleroderma and 'Pseudoscleroderma'." *Speculations in Dermatopathology*. Vol. 2, No. 3, 273-276, Fall 1980.

Caplan, Arnold I. "Cartilage." *Scientific American*. Vol. 251, No. 4, 84-94. Oct. 1984.

Carter, Bayard, Jones, Thomas, Durham, "Invasion of Squamous-Cell Carcinoma of the Cervix Uteri by Endamoeba Histolytica." *Am. J. of Obst. & Gyn*. V. 68, 1607-1610, 1954.

Carter, R. "Primary Amoebic Menigo-Encephalitis, An appraisal of present knowledge." *Transactions of the Royal Society of Tropical Medicine and Hygiene*. Vol. 66, No. 1, 193-213, 1972.

_____, "Primary Amoebic Meningo-Encephalitis: Clinical Pathological and Epidemiological Features of Six Fatal Cases," *The Journal of Pathology and Bacteriology*, Vol. 96, No. 1, 1-25, 1968.

_____, "Sensitivity to Amphotericin B of a *Naegleria* Sp. Isolated from a Case of Primary Amoebic Meningoencephalitis," *Journal Clinical Pathology*, Vol. 22, 470-474, 1969.

_____. "Description of a *Naegleria* sp. Isolated from Two Cases of Primary Amoebic Meningoencephalitis and of the Experimental Pathological Changes Induced by It." *The Journal of Pathology*, Vol. 100, No. 4, 217-244, 1970.

Casemore, David. "Sensitivity of *Hartmannella (Acanthamoeba)* to 5-fluorocytosine, hydroxystilbamidine, and other substances." *J. Clin. Path.* Vol. 23, 649-652, 1970.

—————. "Free-living Amoebae in Home Dialysis Unit." *The Lancet.* Nov. 19, 1078, 1977.

Cathcart, Robert F., III. "Vitamin C, Titrating to Bowel Tolerance, Anascorbemia, and Acute Induced Scurvy," *Medical Hypotheses*, 7: 1359-1376, 1981.

Cerva, K. Novak, C.G. Culbertson. "An Outbreak of Acute, Fatal Amebic Meningoencephalitis." *Am. Journ. of Epidemiology*, Vol. 88, No. 3, 436-444, 1968.

Chapdelaine, Tony. "Preliminary Report on Drug Research Involving *Acanthamoeba* and *Naegleria*". Presented July 14, 1984, at 2nd Physicians and Scientists Meeting of *The Rheumatoid Disease Foundation*, 4 pages, 1984.

Chandar, K., Mair, H., & Mair, N. "Case of Toxoplasma Polymyositis." *Brit. Med. J.*, 158-159, Jan. 20, 1968.

Chang, R.S., & Owens, S. "Patterns of 'Lipovirus' Antibody in Human Populations." *J. Immun.* Vol. 92, 313-319, 1964.

Chang, R. Shihman, I-Hung Pan, Barbara J. Rosenau. "On the Nature of the 'Lipovirus'." *Journ. of Ex. Med.* 124:1153-1166, 1966.

Chari, M.V., B.N. Gadiyar. "A New Drug (MK-910) in the Therapy of Intestinal and Hepatic Amebiasis." *Am. Journ. of Trop. Med. Hyg.* Vol. 19, No. 6, 926-928, 1970.

Charoenlarp, P. Warren, L.G., R.E. Reeves. "Amoebiasis and Intestinal Protozoal Infections." *Trop. Dis. Bul.* Vol. 68, No. 7, 814-819, July 1971.

Chi, L. et al. "Selective Phagocytosis of Nucleated Erythrocytes by Cytotoxic Amebae in Cell Culture." *Science*, Vol. 130, 1763, 1959.

Christ, Helmut W. *Personal Letter and Protocol on Use of Fumaric Acid in Treating Psoriasis, 10 pages, Dec. 16, 1984.*

Chrystal, Ewan J.T., Ronald L. Koch, Martha A. McLafferty, and Peter Goldman. "Relationship Between Metronidazole Metabolism and Bactericidal Activity," *Antimicrobial Agents and Chemotherapy*, 566-573, 1980

Cline, F. Marciano-Cabral, S.G. "Comparison of *Naegleria fowleri* and *Naegleria gruberi* Cultivated in the Same Nutrient Medium. *J. Protozool.*, Vol. 30, No. 2, 387-391, May 1983.

Cox, Eugene C. "Amebic Meningoencephalitis Caused by Acanthamoeba Species in a Four Month Old Child." *Journ. S.C. Med. Assoc.*, Vol. 76, No. 10, 459-462, Oct. 1980.

Coxon, A., C.A. Pallis. "Metronidazole Neuropathy." *J. Neurol. Neurosurg. Psychiat.* 39, 403-405, Apr. 1976.

Craig, Charles. "Observations Upon the Endamebae of the Mouth." *Jour. Infect. Dis.* Vol. 18, 220-239, 1916.

Cranton, E.M., J.P. Frackelton. "Free Radical Pathology in Age-Associated Diseases: Treatment with EDTA Chelation, Nutrition and Antioxidants." *Journ. Holistic Med.* Vol. 6, No. 1, (Reprint) 1-36, Spring/Summer 1984.

Cuckler, A.C., C.M. Malanga, J. Conroy. "Therapeutic Efficacy of New Nitroimidazoles for Experimental Trichomoniasis, Amebiasis, and Trypanosomiasis." *Am. Journ. Trop. Med. Hyg.* Vol. 19, No. 6, 916-925, 1970.

Culbertson, Clyde. "Pathogenic Acanthamoeba (Hartmannella)." *The American Journal of Clinical Pathology.* Vol. 35, No. 3, 195-202, 1961.

—————. "The Pathogenicity of Soil Amebas." *Annual Review of Microbiology.* Vol. 25, 1971, 231-254.

—————. "Soil Ameba Infection." *Am. J. Clin Path.*, Vol. 63, 475-482, 1975.

Culbertson, C., Ensminger, P. & Overton, W. "Hartmannella (Acanthamoeba). Experimental Chronic, Granulomatous Brain Infections, Produced by New Isolates of Low Virulence." *Am. J. Clin. Path.* Vol. 46, 305-314, 1966.

—————. "Amebic Cellulocutaneous Invasion by *Naegleria aerobia* with Generalized Visceral Lesions after Subcutaneous Inoculation: An Experimental Study in Guinea Pigs." *Am. J. Clin. Path.* Vol. 57, 375-386, 1972.

Culbertson, C., Holmes, D. & Overton, W. "*Hartmannella Castellani (Acanthamoeba sp)* Preliminary Report on Experimental Chemotherapy." *The Am. J. of Clin. Path.* Vol. 43, No. 4, 361-364, 1965.

Culbertson, C., Smith, J., Cohen, H. & Minner, J. "Experimental Infection of Mice and Monkeys by Acanthamoeba." *Amer. J. Path.* Vol. 35, 185-197, 1959.

Cunningham, Bruce A. "The Structure and Function of Histocompatibility Antigens." *Scientific American.* 96-107, Oct. 1977.

Cursons, R., T. Brown, E. Keys. "Immunity to Pathogenic Free-living Amoebae." *The Lancet.*, 875-876, Oct. 22, 1977.

Cursons, Ray T.M.., Tim J.. Brown, Elizabeth A. Keys, Kevin M. Moriarty, Desmond Till. "Immunity to Pathogenic Free-living Amoebae: Role of Cell-Mediated Immunity." *Infec. and Immun.* Vol. 29, No. 2, 408-410, Aug. 1980.

Daggett, Pierre-Marc, Thomas A. Nerad. "The Biochemical Identification of Vahlkampfid Amoebae." *J. Protozool.* Vol. 30, No. 1, 126-128, 1983.

Danielson, David A., Marian T. Hannan, Hershel Jack. "Metronidazole and Cancer." *JAMA* Vol. 247, No. 18, 2498-2499, May 14, 1982.

Das, S.R. "Chemotherapy of Experimental Amoebic Meningoencephalitis in Mice Infected with *Naegleria aerobia*." Trans. Roy. Soc. Trop. Med. Hyg., Vol. 65, 106-107, 1971.

Davies, A.H. "Metronidazole in Human Infections with Syphilis." *Brit. J. Vener. Dis.*, Vol. 43, 197-199, 1967.

Davies, A.H., J.A. McFadzean, S. Squires. "Treatment of Vincent's Stomatitis with Metronidazole." *British Med. Journ.*, Vol. i, 1149-1150, May 2, 1964.

Derrick, E. "A Fatal Case of Generalized Amoebiasis Due to a Protozoon Closely Resembling, If Not Identical with, *Iodamoeba Butschlii.*" *Transactions of the Royal Society of Tropical Medicine and Hygiene.* Vol. 42, No. 2, 191-198, 1948.

Dowdle, E.B. "The Immunology of Rheumatoid Arthritis — Role of the Macrophage." *Bylae tot die SA Mediese Tydskjrif.* 14-16, Oct. 19, 1983.

Duma, Richard. "In Vitro Susceptibility of Pathogenic *Naegleria gruberi* to Amphotericin B." *Antimicrobial Agents and Chemotherapy.* 109-111, 1971.

—————. "Primary Amoebic Meningoencephalitis." *Virginia Medical Monthly*, Vol. 96, September, 546-548, 1969.

—————. "Primary Amoebic Meningoencephalitis." *CRC Critical Reviews in Clinical Laboratory Science.* Vol. 3, 163-192, June 1972.

Duma, Ferrell, et al. "Primary Amebic Meningoencephalitis," *The New England Journal of Medicine*, Vol. 281, No. 24, 1315-1323, Dec. 11, 1969.

Duma, R. & Finley, G. "In Vitro Susceptibility of Pathogenic *Naegleria* and *Acanthamoeba* Species to a Variety of Therapeutic Agents." *Antimicrobial Agents and Chemotherapy*, Vol. 10, No. 2, 370-376, Aug. 1976.

Duma, Helwig, & Martinez. "Meningoencephalitis and Brain Abscess Due to a Free-Living Amoeba." *Annals of Internal Medicine.* Vol. 88, 468-473, 1978.

Duma, Richard J., William I. Rosenblum, Read F. McGehee, Muriel M. Jones, E. Clifford Nelson. "Primary Amoebic Meningoencephalitis Caused by *Naegleria*," *Annals of Internal Medicine*, Vol. 74, 861-869, 1971.

Dunnebacke, Thelma H., Robley C. Williams. "A Reinterpretation of the Nature of 'Lipovirus' Cytopathogenicity," *Proceedings National Academy of Science*, Vol. 57, 1967.

Edelman, Gerald M. "The Structure and Function of Antibodies." *Scientific American*, 34-42, 1970.

Edwards, J.H., A.J. Griffiths, J. Mullins. "Protozoa as Sources of Antigen in 'Humidifier Fever'." *Nature*, Vol. 264, 438-439, Dec. 2, 1976.

Efron, Edith. "The Big Cancer Lie." *The American Spectator.* Vol. 17, No. 3, 10-17, March 1984.

Eldridge, A. & Tobin, J. "'Ryan Virus'." *Brit. Med. J.*, 299, Feb. 4, 1967.

Evers, Ray. "Method and Composition for Treating Arteriosclerosis." *United States Patent 4,167,562.* Pages 4, Sept. 11, 1979.

Eyles, D., et al. "A Study of *Endamoeba Histolytica* and Other Intestinal Parasites in a Rural West Tennessee Community." *The American Journal of Tropical Medicine and Hygiene*, Vol. 2, 173-190, 1953.

Ferguson, K. & Anderson, R. "Amebic Liver Abscess in Service Personnel." *Gastroenterology.* Vol. 8, 332-342, 1947.

Ferrante, A. B. Rowan-Kelly, Y.H. Thong. "*In Vitro* Sensitivity of Virulent *Acanthamoeba culbertsoni* to a Variety of Drugs and Antibiotics." *Int. Journ. Parasit.*, Vol. 14, No. 1, 53-56, 1984.

Forre, O., E. Munthe, E. Kass. "Side-Effects and Autoimmunogenicity of D-Penicillamine Treatment in Rheumatic Diseases." *Advances in Inflammation Research*, Vol. 6, 251-257, 1984.

Fowler, M. & Carter, R.F. "Acute Pyogenic Meningitis Probably Due to *Acanthamoeba* sp.: a Preliminary Report." *British Medical Journal*, 740-742, September 25, 1965.

Frye, W. et al. "Antibiotics in the Treatment of Acute Amoebic Dysentery." *Annals New York Academy Sciences*, 1104-1113, 1952.

Fulford, S.G. Bradley, F. Marciano-Cabral, "Cytopathogenticity of *Naegleria fowleri*, for Cultured Rat Neuroblastoma Cells" Unpublished paper, Dept. Microbiology and Immun., Virginia Commonwealth University, Richmond, VA 23298, 20 pages, no date.

Garcia-Laverde, A. & De Bonilla, L. "Clinical Trials with Metronidazole in Human Balantidiasis." *Am. J. Trop. Med. & Hyg.* Vol. 24, No. 5, 781-783, 1975.

Goldman, Peter. "Metronidazole: Proven Benefits and Potential Risks." *Johns Hopkins Med. Journ.* 147, 1-9, 1980.

Goobar, J. "Joint Symptoms in Giardiasis." *The Lancet.* 1010-1011, May 7, 1977.

Griffin, Joe L. "Temperature Tolerance of Pathogenic and Nonpathogenic Free-Living Amoebas." *Science.* Vol. 178, Nov. 24, 1972.

Grunnet, Margaret L., George H. Cannon, James P. Kushner. "Fulminant Amebic Meningoencephalitis due to *Acanthamoeba*." *Neurology.* (Ny)31, 174-177, Feb. 1981.

Gunby, Phil, "Allopurinol Treatment for Protozoan Infections?" *Journal of American Medical Association*, Vol. 240, No. 18, Oct. 27, 1978, 1941-1942.

Gullett, J., John Mills, Keith Hadley, Benjamin Podemski, Lawrence Pitts, Robert Gelber. "Disseminated Granulomatous Infection Presenting as an Unusual Skin Lesion." *The American Journal of Medicine*, Vol. 67, 891-896, Nov. 1979.

Han, Jang H., Kwang H. Jeon. "Isolation and Partial Characterization of Two Plasmid Deoxyribonucleic Acids from Endosymbiotic Bacteria of *Amoeba proteus*". *Journ. Bact.* 1466-1469, Mar. 1980.

Hamilton, Delores M. Elliott. "Combined Activity of Amphotericin B and 5-Fluorocytosine against *Cryptococcus neoformans* in Vitro and in Vivo in Mice." *Journ. of Infect. Dis.*, Vol. 131, No. 2, 129-137., Feb. 1975.

Harkness, J.A.L., A.J. Griffin, I. Heinrich, T. Gibson and R. Grahame. "A Double-Blind Comparative Study of Metronidazole and Placebo in Rheumatoid Arthritis." *Rheumatology and Rehabilitation*, 21, 231-234, 1982.

Hines, Laurence. "Endameba Histolytica in Seminal Fluid in a Case of Amebic Dysentery." *J.A.M.A.*, Vol. 81, No. 4, 274-275, 1923.

Hoffmann, E., C. Garcia, J. Lunseth, P. McGarry, J. Coover. "A Case of Primary Amebic Meningoencephalitis." *Am. J. Trop. Med. & Hyg.*, Vol. 27 No. 1, 29-38, 1978.

Hunter, William. "Discussion on Oral Sepsis as a Cause of Disease in Relation to General Medicine." *The British Medical Journal.* Nov. 19, 1358-1363, 1904.

Husain, M. & Mohan Rao, V. "Aminotransferase Activity of Hartmanella (Culbertson strain A-1) Grown Axenically." *J. Gen. Microbiology*, Vol. 56, 379-386, 1969.

Imam, S.A., G.P. Dutta, S.C. Agarwala. "Inhibition of Excystment of *Schizopyrenus russelli* Cysts in the Presence of Emetine and Its Cysticidal Effect in Conjunction with Sodium Lauryl Sulphate." *J. Gen. Microbiol.*, Vol. 51, 171-221, 1968.

Jakovljevich, R., B. Talis. "Recovery of Hartmannelloid Ameba in the Purulent Discharge from a Human Ear." *J. Protozol.*, Vol. 16, 36, 1969.

Jahnes, W., Harold M. Fullmer, and C.P. Li, et al. "Free Living Amoebae as Contaminants in Monkey Kidney Tissue Culture." *Proc. Soc. Exp. Biol. Med.*, Vol. 96, 484-488, 1957.

Jeon, Kwang W. "Integration of Bacterial Endosymbionts in Amoebae." *International Rev. of Cytology*, Supplement 14, 29-47, 1983.

——————, I. Joan Lorch. "The Formation of Vacuole Membranes in the Presence and Absence of Cell Nucleus in Amoebae." *Exp. Cell Res.* Reprint: 141, 351-356, 1982.

Johnstone, T. "Primary Amebic Meningoencephalitis." *Personal Letter: Swimming pools*: From Johnstone to J.W. Shaw, Env. Hlth. Eng., Env. Hlth. Srv., Lcl. Brd. Hlth., Edmonton, Alberta, Canada, (2 pp.), Feb. 20, 1980.

Jones, D., Visvesvara, G., & Robinson, N. "*Acanthamoeba polyphaga* Keratitis and *Acanthamoeba* Uveitis Associated with Fatal Meningoencephalitis." *Trans. of the Opthal. Soc. of the United Kingdom*, Vol. 93, 221-232, 1975.

Jubb, R. "Non-steroidal Anti-inflammatory Drugs and Articular Cartilage," Publication Unknown. 6-8.

Kenney, Michael. "The Micro-Kolmer Complement Fixation Test in Routine Screening for Soil Ameba Infection." *Health Laboratory Science*, Vol. 8, No. 1, 5-10, 1971.

Kerkering, Thomas M., Pauline M. Schwartz, Ana Espinel-Ingroff, Paul J. Turek, Robert B. Diasio. "5-Fluorocytosine Susceptibility of Pathogenic Fungi in the Presence of Allopurinol: Potential for Improving the Therapeutic Index of 5-Fluorocytosine," *Antimicrobial Agents and Chemotherapy*, Vol. 24, No. 3, 448-449, Sept. 1983.

Kernohan, J., Magath, T., & Schloss, G. "Granuloma of Brain Probably Due to Endolimax Williamsi (Iodamoeba Butschlii)." *Archives of Pathology.* Vol. 70, 576-580, 1960.

Key, Samuel III, W. Richard Green, Eddy Willaert, Ann R. Stevens, Samuel N. Key, Jr. "Keratitis Due to *Acanthamoeba castellani*." *Archives of Opthalmology*, Vol. 98, 475-479, March 1980.

Kingston, D. & Warhurst, D. "Isolation of Amoeba from the Air." *Jour. of Medical Microbiology*, Vol. 2, 27-36, 1969.

Kishore, V., D.W. Roberts, J.B. Barnett, J.R.J. Sorenson. "Effect of Nutritional Copper Deficiency on Adjuvant Arthritis and Immunocompetence in the Rat." *Agents and Actions*, Vol. 14, 2, 275-282, 1984.

Kishore, Neal Latman, Randy G. Dotson, John R.J. Sorenson. "Effect of Nutritional Copper Deficiency on the Development of Adjuvant Arthritis in the Rat." *Trace Substances in Environmental Health*, XVI, 291-299, 1982.

Klatskin, Gerald. "Amebiasis of the Liver: Classification, Diagnosis and Treatment." *Ann. Int. Med.* Vol. 25, 601-631, 1946.

Koch, Ronald L., Ewan J.T. Chrystal, Bernard B. Beaulieu, Jr. Peter Goldman. "Acetamide — A Metabolite of Metronidazole Formed by the Intestinal Flora," *Biochemical Pharm.*, Vol. 28, 3611-3615, 1979.

131

Kofoid, Boyers & Swezy. "The Cytology of Endamoeba Gingivalis (Gros) Brumpt Compared With That of E. Dysenteriae With Special Reference to the Determination of the Amoebas in Bone Marrow in Arthritis Deformans of Ely's Second Type." *Univ. of Calif. Publ. in Zoology.* Vol. 26, No. 9, 165-198, 1924.

_____. "Endameba Dysenteriae in the Lymph Glands of Man in Hodgkin's Disease." *Univ. of Calif. Publ. in Zoology.* Vol. 20, No. 12, 309-312, 1922.

_____. "Mitosis in Endamoeba Dysenteriae in The Bone Marrow in Arthritis Deformans." *Univ. of Calif. Publ. in Zoology.* Vol. 20, No. 11, 301-307, 1922.

_____. "Occurrence of Endamoeba Dysenteriae in the Lesions of Hodgkin's Disease." *J.A.M.A.* Vol. 78, No. 21, 1604-1607, 1922.

_____. "On the Free, Encysted & Budding Stages of Councilmania Lafleuri, a Parasitic Amoeba of the Human Intestine." *Univ. of Calif. Publ. in Zoology.* Vol. 20, No. 7, 169-198, June 23, 1921.

_____. "On the Prevalence of Carriers of Endamoeba Dysenteriae Among Soldiers Returned from Overseas Service." *Am. Jour. Trop. Med.* Vol i, No. 1, 41-48, Jan. 1921.

_____. "Karyamoeba falcata, a New Amoeba from the Human Intestinal Tract." *Univ. of Calif. Publ. in Zoology.* Vol. 26, No. 11, 221-242, 1924.

Kofoid, Swezy & Boyers. "The Coexistence of Hodgkin's Disease and Amebiasis." *J.A.M.A.* Vol. 78, 532, 1922.

_____. "The Coexistence of Hodgkin's Disease and Amebiasis." *J.A.M.A.* Vol. 78, No. 15, 1147, 1922.

_____. "Endamoeba Dystenteriae — in the Lymph Glands of Man in Hodgkin's Disease, *Univ. of Cal. Pub. in Zoo.*, Vol. 20, No. 12, pp. 390-312, April 21, 1922.

Kofoid, Charles A.; Olive Swezy. "Amebiasis of the Bones," *Jour. A.M.A.* 1602-1607, May 27, 1922.

Kofoid, C. & Wagener, E. "Studies of the Effects of Certain Drugs Upon Endamoeba Dysenteriae *in Vitro.*" *Univ. of Cal. Publ. in Zool.* Vol. 28, No. 6, 155-166, 1925.

Kurtz, Theodore W., R. Curtis Morris, Jr. "Dietary Chloride as a Determinant of 'Sodium-Dependent' Hypertension." *Science.* Vol. 222, 1139-1141, Sept. 20, 1983.

Leder, Philip. "The Genetics of Antibody Diversity." *Scientific American.* 102-115, May 1982.

Lee, C.W., R.A. Lewis, E.J. Corey, K.F. Austen. "Human Biology and Immunoreactivity of Leukotrienes." *Advances in Inflammation Research.* Vol. 6, 219-225, 1984.

Leipzig, L.J., A.J. Boyle, D.S. McCann. "Case Histories of Rheumatoid Arthritis Treated with Sodium or Magnesium EDTA." *J. Chron. Dis.* Vol. 22, 553-563, 1970.

Levine, Stephen A., "Oxidants/Anti-Oxidants and Chemical Hypersensitivities (Part One)." *Int. Journ. Biosocial Res.* Vol. 4, No. 1, 51-54, 1983.

_____. "Oxidants/Anti-Oxidants and Chemical Hypersensitivities (Part Two)." *Int. Journ. Biosocial Res.* Vol. 4, No. 2, 102-105, 1983.

Levine, Stephen A., Jay Parker. "Selenium and Human Chemical Hypersensitivities: Preliminary Findings." *Int. Journ. Biosocial Res.* Vol. 3, No. 1, 44-47, 1982.

Levine, Stephen A., Jeffrey H. Reinhardt. "Biochemical-Pathology Initiated by Free Radicals, Oxidant Chemicals and Therapeutic Drugs in the Etiology of Chemical Hypersensitivity Disease." *Journ. Orthomolecular Psy.* Third Quarter, Vol. 12, No. 3, 166-183, 1983.

Liu, Chien, Patricia Rodina. "Immunofluorescent Studies of Human Cell Cultures and Chick Embryos Inoculated with the Ameboid Cell — 'Lipovirus' Complex." *J. Exp. Med.* 124:1167, 1966.

Lorch, I. Joan, Kwang W. Jeon. "Resuscitation of Amebae Deprived of Essential Symbiotes: Micrurgical Studies." *Jour. Protozool.* 27(4) 423-426, 1980.

_____. "Nuclear Lethal Effect and Nucleocytoplasmic Incompatibility Induced by Endosymbionts in *Amoeba proteus*." *Jour. Protozool.* (29)3 468-470, 1982.

_____. "Rapid Induction of Cellular Strain Specificity by Newly Acquired Cytoplasmic Components in Amoebas." *Science.* Vol. 211, 949-951, Feb. 27, 1981.

Luna, R. Pacheco. "Acute Iritis Developed after Amebic Dysentery." *Am. J. Opthal.* 658-660, Sept. 1918.

Lund, O.E., F.H. Stefani, W. Dechant. "Amoebic Keratitis: A Clinicopathological Case Report." *Brit. Journ. Opth.* 62, 373-375, 1978.

Lynch, Kenneth. "An Ameba in Suppurative and Hyperplastic Osteoperiostitis of Inferior Maxilla." *J.A.M.A.* Vol. 65, No. 24, 2077, 1915.

Lyons, Trevor. *Oral Amoebiasis. Dentofacts.* Vol. IX, No. 7, 12 pages, (Also Research Program, Patient's Information Literature — Periodontal (Pyorrhea) Disease and Oral Parasites: pages 1-7.), July 1980.

Lyons, Thomas, III, Thomas & Kapur, Ramesh. "Limax Amoebae in Public Swimming Pools of Albany, Schenectady, and Rensselaer Counties, New York: Their Concentration, Correlations, and Significance." *Applied and Environmental Microbiology,* Vol. 33, No. 3, 551-555, March 1977.

Mahomedy, Y.M. "Treatment of Rheumatoid Arthritis," *S. Afr. Jour. of Cont. Medical Ed.*, 12, Deel 1, Nov. 1983.

Marciano-Cabral, F.M., S.G. Bradley. "Cytopathogenicity of *Naegleria gruberi* for Rat Neuroblastoma Cell Cultures," *Inf. and Imm.*, Vol. 35, No. 3, 1139-1141, Mar. 1982.

Marciano-Cabral, F.M., M. Patterson, D.T. John, S.G. Bradley, "Cytopathogenicity of *Naegleria fowleri* and *Naegleria gruberi* for Established Mammalian Cell Cultures, *J. Parasitol.* 68(6) 1110-1116, 1982.

Marino, Joseph. *"Amplification of Primary Amebic Meningoencephalitis." The Journal of Pediatrics,* Vol. 86, No. 1, 160-161, Jan. 1975.

Markowitz, Sheldon, M. Thomas Sobieski, A. Julio Martinez, Richard J. Duma. "Experimental Infections in Mice Pretreated with Methylprednisolone or Tetracycline." *Am. Journ. Path.* Vol. 92 No. 3, 733-743, Sept. 1978.

Martin, Wayne. "The Beriberi Analogy to Myocardial Infarction", *Medical Hypothesis,* 10:185-198, 1983.

_____. "Combined Role of Atheroma, Cholesterol, Platelets, the Endothelium and Fibrin in Heart Attacks and Strokes, PO Box 1133, Fairhope, AL 36532, 18 pages, no date.

_____. "Do We Get Too Much Iron," *Medical Hypothesis,* 13, 119-121, 1984

_____. "Talk Before the Seattle Chapter of the International Association of Cancer Victims and Friends, 14 pages, Sept. 23, 1984.

Martinez, Julio. "Is *Acanthamoeba* Encephalitis an Opportunistic Infection?" *Neurology,* Vol. 30, 567-574, June 1980.

_____. "Acanthamoebiasis and Immunosuppression." *Journal of Neuropathology and Experimental Neurology,* Vol. 41, No. 5, 548-557, Sept. 1982.

132

Martinez, A. Julio, Richard J. Duma, E. Clifford Nelson, Frank L. Moretta. "Experimental Naegleria Meningoencephalitis in Mice." *Laboratory Investigation*. Vol. 29, No. 2, 121-133, 1973.

Martinez, A. Julio, Carlos A. Garcia, Meredith Halks-Miller, Rafael Arce-Vela. "Granulomatous Amebic Encephalitis Presenting as a Cerebral Mass Lesion." *Acta Neuropathol*. (Berl.) 51, 85-91, 1980.

Martinez, A. Julio, Sheldon M. Markowitz, Richard J. Duma. "Experimental Pneumonitis and Encephalitis Caused by *Acanthamoeba* in Mice: Pathogenesis and Ultrastructural Features." *J. Inf. Dis*. Vol. 131, No. 6, 692-699. June 1975.

Martinez, A. Julio, Cirilo Sotelo-Avila, Hilda Alcala, Eddy Willaert. "Granulomatous Encephalitis, Intracranial Arteritis, and Mycotic Aneurysm Due to a Free-Living Ameba." *Acta Neuropathol*. (Berl.) 49, 7-12, 1980.

Martinez, A. Julio, Cirilo Sotelo-Avila, Jorge Garcia-Tamayo, Juan Takano Moron, Eddy Willaert, William P. Stamm. "Meningoencephalitis Due to Acanthamoeba SP." *Acta Neuropathologica*, Vol. 37, 183-191, 1977.

Martinez, Garcia, et al. "Granulomatous Amebic Encephalitis Presenting as a Cerebral Mass Lesion." *Acta Neuropathologica*. Vol. 51, 85-91, 1980.

McCowen, M. et al. "The Effects of Erythromycin (Ilotycin, Lilly) Against Certain Parasitic Organisms." *The Am. J. of Trop. Med. & Hyg.*, Vol. 2, 212-218, 1953.

McFadzean, et al. "The Interactions of Metronidazole and Micro-organisms." *The Indian Practitioner*, 623-624, Oct. 1968.

McMillan, Bruce. "The Inhibition of Leptomonads of the Genus *Leishmania* in Culture by Antifungal Antibiotics." *Ann. Trop. Med. & Parasit.*, Vol. 54, 293-299, 1960.

McNeill, R. & Moraes-Ruehsen, M. "Ameba Trophozoites in Cervico-Vaginal Smear of a Patient Using an Intrauterine Device." *Acta Cytologica*, Vol. 22, No. 2, 91-92, 1978.

Meleney, H., Bishop, E. & Leathers, W. "Investigations of *Endamoeba Histolytica* and Other Intestinal Protozoa in Tennessee" *Am. J. Hyg.* Vol. 16, 523-539, 1932.

Miller, Julie Ann. "Antibodies for Sale." *Science News*. Vol. 123, 296-298, May 7, 1983.

Mills, Lloyd. "Amoebic Iritis Occurring in the Course of Non-dysenteric Amebiasis." *Archives of Opthalmology* Vol. 52, No. 6, 525-545, 1923.

Mitelman, Felix, Bodil Strombeck, Bo Ursing. "No Cytogenetic Effect of Metronidazole." *Lancet*. 1249-50, June 7, 1980.

Milstein, Cesar. "Monoclonal Antibodies." *Scientific American*. 66-74, October 1980.

Moore, Alice E., John Hlinka. "Hartmanella sp. (acanthamoeba) as a Tissue Culture Contaminant," *J. of the Natl. Cancer Inst.*, Vol. 40, No. 3, March 1968.

Morring, Kathy L., W.G. Sorenson, Michael D. Attfield. "Sampling for Airborne Fungi: A Statistical Comparison of Media," *Am. Ind. Hyg. Assoc. J.* 449(9) 662-664, Sept. 1983.

Moss, Ralph W. "The Politics of Cancer: The Promise of Hydrazine Sulfate." *Penthouse*. Jan. 1983.

Most, H. & Van Assendelft, F. "Treatment of Amoebiasis with Terramycin." *Annals New York Academy Sciences*, 1114-1117, 1952.

Nagington, J., P.G. Watson, T.J. Playfair, J. McGill, Barrie R. Jones, A.D. McG. Steele. "Amoebic Infection of the Eye." *The Lancet*. 1537-1540, Dec. 28, 1974.

Nagington, J. & Smith, D. "Pontiac Fever and Amoebae." *The Lancet*. 1241, Dec. 6, 1980.

Nakamura, Mitsuru, et al. "Drug Effects on the Metabolism of *Endamoeba histolytica; In vitro* and *In vivo* Tests of Synergism." *The Am. J. of Trop. Med. & Hyg.*, Vol. 2, 206-211, 1953.

Neff, Robert J. "Purification, Axenic Cultivation, and Description of a Soil Amoeba, *Acanthamoeba* sp." *J. Protozool*. 4, 176-182, 176-182, 1957.

Nerad, Thomas A., Govinda Visvesvara, Pierre-Marc Daggett. "Chemically Defined Meda for the Cultivation of *Naegleria*: Pathogenic and High Temperature Tolerant Species." *J. Protozool*. Vol. 30, No. 2, 383-387, 1983.

Notkins, Abner Louis, Hilary Koprowski. "How the Immune Response to a Virus Can Cause Disease." *Scientific American*. 22-31, 1973.

Oser, B. & Hosler, R. "Amebiasis with Complicating Encephalitis Probably Due to Entamoeba Histolytica." *The Ohio State Medical Journal*, Vol. 56, 1502-1503, 1960.

Otterness, Ivan G. "Clotrimazole and Rheumatoid Arthritis." *The Lancet*. 148, Jan. 17, 1976.

Oye, Robert K., Martin F. Shapiro. "Reporting Results From Chemotherapy Trials," *JAMA*, Vol. 252, No. 19, 2722-2724, Nov. 16, 1984.

Page, Frederick. "Taxonomic and Ecological Distribution of Potentially Pathogenic Free-Living Amoebae." *Journ. of Para.*, Vol. 56, No. 4, Sec. II, Part 1, 257-258, 1970.

_____. "Taxonomic Criteria for Limax Amoebae, with Descriptions of 3 New Species of *Hartmannella* and 3 of *Vahlkampfia*." *Journal of Protozoology* Vol. 14, No. 3, 1967, 499-521.

_____. "Redefinition of the Genus *Acanthamoeba* with Descriptions of Three Species." *Journal of Protozoology*. Vol. 14, No. 4, 1967, 709-724.

_____. Resumes of Contributions. *Journal of Parasitology*, Vol. 56, No. 4, Section II, Part I, August, 1970, 257-258.

Panush, Richard S.; Richard Yonker. "Rheumatoid Arthritis: Disease Outside the Joints." *Diagnosis*. 103-108, May 1983.

Patterson, T.W. Woodworth, F. Marciano-Cabral. "Ultrastructure of *Naegleria fowleri* Enflagellation," *Journ. Bacter.* J Vol. 147, No. 1, p. 217-226, Jul. 1981.

Parelkar, W.P. Stamm, K.R. Hill. "Indirect Immunofluorescent Staining of Entamoeba Histolytica in Tissues." *The Lancet*. 212-213, Jan. 30, 1971.

Patras, Dorothy & Andujar, John. "Meningoencephalitis due to Hartmannella (Acanthamoeba)." *The Am. J. of Clin. Path*. Vol. 46, No. 2, 226-233, 1966.

Patterson, M., T.W. Woodworth, F., Marciano-Cabral, S.G. Bradley. "Ultrastructure of *Naegleria fowleri* Enflagellation." *Journ. Bacter*. 217-226, Vol. 147, No. 1, July 1981.

Pennington, J., Block, E. & Reynolds, H. "5-Fluorocytosine and Amphotericin B in Bronchial Secretions." *Antimicrobial Agents and Chemotherapy*, Vol. 6, No. 3, Sept. 1974, 324-326.

Pereira, M. et al. "Ryan Virus: a Possible New Human Pathogen." *British Medical Journal*, Jan. 15, 1966, 130-132.

Platt, Philip N. "Examination of Synovial Fluid," *Clinics in Rheumatic Dis.*, Vol. 9, No. 1, 51-67, Apr. 1983.

Powell, S.J., A.J. Wilmot, I. MacLeon, R. Elsdon-Dew. "Metronidazole in Amoebic Dysentery and Amoebic Liver Abscess." *The Lancet*, Dec. 17, 1966, 1329-1331.

Prasad, B.N. "*In vitro* Effect of Drugs Against Pathogenic and Non-Pathogenic Free-Living Amoebae and on Anaerobic Amoebae." *Indian Journal of Experimental Biology*, Vol. 10, Jan. 1972, 43-45.

Prata, Aluizio. "Treatment of Kala-azar with Amphotericin B." *Transactions of the Royal Society of Tropical Medicine and Hygiene*, Vol. 57, No. 4, July 1963, 266-268.

Pringle, H. L., S.G. Bradley, L.S. Harris. "Susceptibility of *Naegleria fowleri* to Delta⁹-Tetrahydrocannabinol, *Antimicrobial Agents and Chemotherapy*, Vol. 16, No. 5, 674-679, Nov. 1979.

Pybus, Paul K. "Anti-amoebic Drugs in Rheumatoid Arthritis." *SA Mediese Tydskrif.* Deel 63, Jan. 8, 1983.
_____. "Easy Control of the Painful and Stiff Hand." *Unpublished Paper.* March 27, 1984.
_____. "Metronidazole in Rheumatoid Arthritis." *SA Medical Jour.* Vol. 65, 454, Mar. 24, 1984.
_____. "Metronidazole in Rheumatoid Arthritis." *SA Mediese Tydskrif.* 261-262, Feb. 20, 1982.
_____. "Nerve Stabilisation." *British Medical Acupuncture Soc. Journ.* 16-17, June 1984.
_____. "Tender Spots Around the Osteo-Arthritic Knee," *SA Med. Journ.* Vol. 64, 270, Aug. 20, 1983.
Rappaport, E., Rossien, A. & Rosenblum, L. "Arthritis Due to Intestinal Amebiasis." *Ann. Int. Med.* Vol. 34, 1951, 1224-1231.
Reilly, M.F., M.K. Bradley, S.G. Bradley. "Agglutination of *Naegleria fowleri* by Human Serum, *Proc. Soc. for Exp. Biology and Med.* 17-, 209-212, 1982.
_____, F. Marciano-Cabral, D.W. Bradley, S.G. Bradley. "Agglutination of *Naegleria fowleri* and *Naegleria gruberi* by Antibodies in Human Serum, *Journ. Clin. Microbiology,* Vol. 17, No. 4, 576-581, Apr. 1983.
Renforth, William, M.D. "Metronidazole Cures Rheumatoid Arthritis." *Unpublished Paper.* Sept. 30, 1977.
Ringsted, Jorgen, B. Val Jager, Dongsoo Suk, Govinda S. Visvesvara. "Probable Acanthamoeba Meningoencephalitis in a Korean Child." *Am. J. Clin. Path.,* Vol. 66, 1976, 723-730.
Robert, Victor, & Rorke, Lucy. "Primary Amebic Encephalitis, Probably from *Acanthamoeba*." *Annals of Internal Medicine,* Vol. 79, 1973, 174-179.
Robinson, Harry. "General Pharmacology of Antibiotics." *Annals N.Y. Acad. Sci.,* Vol. 55, 1952, 970-982.
Rollo, Ian M. "Drugs Used in the Chemotherapy of Amebiasis." Chapter 46. (Metronidazole, 8-Hydroxyquinolines, Emetine, Dehydroemetine, Chloroquine, Diloxanide Furoate). *The Pharmocological Basis of Therapeutics.* Weinstein Publ. N.Y., 1061, 1980.
_____. "Miscellaneous Drugs Used in the Treatment of Protozoal Infections." Chapter 47, (Suramin, Pentamidine, Melarsoprol, Other Arsenicals, Sodium Stibogluconate, Metronidazole, Nifurtimox, Quinacrine). (Ed. L.S. Goodman) *Ibid.* 1070-1079, 1980.
Rothrock, John F., Harvey W. Buchsbaum. "Primary Amebic Meningoencephalitis." *JAMA* Vol. 243, No. 22, 2329-2330, June 13, 1980.
Rowbotham, T. "Pontiac Fever Explained?" *The Lancet.* Nov. 1, 1980, 969.
_____. "Pontiac Fever, Amoebae, and Legionellae." *The Lancet,* Jan. 3, 1981.
Rowland, Lewis & Greer, Melvin. "Toxoplasmic polymyositis." *Neurology.* Vol. 11, No. 5, 1961, 367-370.
Salem, Hassan Hilmy, Hassan Abd Rabbo. "Clinical Trials with Dehydroemetine Dihydrochloride in the Treatment of Acute Amoebiasis." *J. Trop. Med. Hyg.* Vol. 67, 137-141, June 1964.
Sargeaunt, P. & Lumsden, W. "*In Vitro* Sensitivity of *Entamoeba histolytica* to furazolidone and iodochlorhydroxyquin, separate and combined." *Trans. of the Roy. Soc. Trop. Med. Hyg.* Vol. 70, No. 1, 1976, 54-56.
Saltztein, Sidney, Lauren V. Ackerman. "Lymphadenopathy Induced by Anticonvulsant Drugs and Mimicking Clinically and Pathologically Malignant Lymphomas." *Cancer* N.Y. 12, 164-182, 1959.
Sawyer, Phillis R., R.N. Brogden, R.M. Pinder, T.M. Speight, G.S. Avery. "Clotrimazole: A Review of its Antifungal Activity and Therapeutic Efficacy." *Drugs* 9:424-447, 1975.
Schuster, F. & Rechthand, E. "In Vitro Effects of Amphotericin B on Growth and Ultrastructure of the Amoeboflagellates *Naegleria gruberi* and *Naegleria fowleri*." *Antimicrobial Agents and Chemotherapy,* Vol. 8, No. 5, 1975, 591-605.
Searle. "Tumorigenic of Metronidazole." *Searle Research and Development, Division of G.D. Searle & Co., 4901 Searle Parkway, Skokie, Illinois 60077.* Personal Letter to Wayne Martin, August 27, 1984. 2 pages, August 27, 1984.
Searle. "Ineffectiveness of Metronidazole for RD." *Searle Research and Development, Division of G.D. Searle & Co., 4901 Searle Parkway, Skokie, Illinois 60077.* Personal Letter to Edmund Talanda, M.D. August 22, 1984 2 pages, August 22, 1984.
Shookhoff, H. & Sterman, M. "Treatment of Amoebiasis with Aureomycin and Bacitracin." *Annals New York Academy Sciences,* 1952, 1125-1132.
Shumaker, Jay B., George R. Healy, Donna English, Myron Schultz, Frederick C. Page. "*Naegleria gruberi*: Isolation from Nasal Swab of a Healthy Individual." *The Lancet.* 602-603, Sept. 11, 1971.
Sigel, Helmut. "Metal Ions in Biological Systems." *Inorganic Drugs in Deficiency and Disease.* Vol. 14, 77-124, 1982.
Simoons, J.R.A. "Product Development Under F.D.A. Regulations in the U.S.A." *Overdruk uit Pharmaceutisch.* Weeblad No. 18, 293-301, 1972.
_____. "Selection of Clotrimazole for Clinical Evaluation." pages 5, *Personal Letter to Rheumatoid Disease Board Members and Scientific Advisory Committee,* July 23, 1984.
Simpson, Robert W., Laurel McGinty, Lee Simon, Carol A. Smith, Carl W. Godzeski, Robert J. Boyd. "Association of Parvoviruses with Rheumatoid Arthritis of Humans." *Science,* Mar. 30, 1984, 1425-1428.
Smith, A., Middleton, W., & Barrett, M. "The Tonsils as a Habitat of Oral Endamebas." *J.A.M.A.* Vol. 63, No. 20, 1914, 1746-1749.
Soltys, M.A., P.T.K. Woo. "An Amoeba-Agglutination Test with *Acanthamoeba (Hartmanella)*." *Trans. Roy. Soc. Trop. Med. Hyg.,* Vol. 63, 426, 1969.
Soren, Arnold, Theodore R. Waugh. "The Giant Cells in the Syunovial Membrane," *Annals of the Rheum. Dis.* 40, 496-500, 1981.
Sorenson, John R. "Copper Aspirinate, a More Potent Antiinflammatory and Antiulcer Agent." Reprint: John R. Sorenson, College of Pharmacy, Univ. of Arkansas for Medical Sciences, 7-22, date unknown.
_____. "Use of Copper Complexes Offers a Physiologic Approach to Treatment of Chronic Diseases." *In Press.* Department of Medicinal Chemistry, Univ. Arkansas College of Pharmacy, 4301 W. Markham, Little Rock, Arkansas 72205.
Sorenson, John R.J., Larry W. Oberley, Rosalie K. Crouch, Thomas W. Kensler, Vimal Kishore, Susan W.C. Leuthauser, Terry D. Oberley, Abbas Pezeshk. "Pharmacologic Activities of Copper Compounds in Chronic Diseases." *Biological Trace Element Research.* 5, 257-273, 1983.
Sorenson, John R.J., Vimal Kishore, Abbas Pezeshk, Larry W. Oberley, Susan W.C. Leuthauser, Terry D. Oberley. "Copper Complexes: A Physiological Approach to the Treatment of 'Inflammatory Diseases'." *Inorganica Chimica Acta.* 91, 285-294, 1984.
Sorenson, John R.J., Thomas M. Rolniak, Louis W. Chang. "Preliminary Chronic Toxicity Study of Copper Aspirinate." *Inorganica Chimca Acta.* 91 L31-L34, 1984.
Sorenson, John R.J., Vimal Kishore. "Antirheumatic Activity of Copper Complexes." *Trace Elements in Medicine.* In press. Presented Oslo Rheumatism Hospital, Oslo, Norway, 15 pages, Oct. 20, 1983.
Sotelo-Avila, C., Taylor, F., & Ewing, C. "Primary Amebic Meningoencephalitis in a Healthy 7-Year-Old Boy." *Journal of Pediatrics,* Vol. 85, No. 1, July, 1974, 131-136.
Spellberg, M. & Zivin, S. "Amebiasis in Veterans of World War II with Special Emphasis on Extra-Intestinal Complications, Including a Case of Amebic Cerebellar Abscess." *Gastroenterology* Vol. 10, No. 3, 1948, 452-473.
Stamm, W. — Abstracts 1434 & 1435. *Tropical Diseases Bulletin,* Vol. 68, No. 7, July 1971, 816-817.
Stamm, W., Ashley, M. & Bell, K. "The Value of Amoebic Serology in an Area of Low Endemicity." *Trans. of the Roy. Soc. of Trop. Med. & Hyg.* Vol. 70, No. 1, 1976, 49-53.

134

Steinberg, Sarah. "Cancer and Cuisine." *Science News.* Vol. 124, No. 14, 217, Oct. 1, 1983.

Stevens, A., W. O'Dell. "In Vitro and In Vivo Activity of 5-Fluorocytosine on *Acanthamoeba.*" *Antimicrobial Agents and Chemotherapy,* Vol. 6, No. 3, 282-289.Sept. 1974.

Stevens, Stanford T. Shulman, Thomas A. Lansen, M.J. Chichon, E. Willaert. "Primary Amoebic Meningoencephalitis: A Report of Two Cases and Antibiotic and Immunologic Studies." *Journ. Infec. Dis.* 143, No. 2, 193-199, Feb. 1981.

Stevens, A.R., E. Willaert. "Drug Sensitivity and Resistance of Four *Acanthamoeba* species." *Trans. Roy. Soc. Trop. Med. Hyg.* Vol. 74, No. 6, 806-808, 1980.

Swezy, Olive. "Mitosis in the Encysted Stages of Endamoeba Coli(Loesch)." *Univ. of Calif. Publications in Zoology.* Vol. 20, No. 13, 1922, 313-332.

Thong, Y. et al. "Growth inhibition of Naegleria Fowleri by Tetracycline, Rifamycin, and Miconazole." *The Lancet.* Oct. 22, 1977, 876.

Tongeren, J.H.M. "Rheumatoid-Factor-Like Globulins and Tropical Parasitic Infections." *The Lancet.* 1266, June 4, 1966.

Torres, Elena Fentanes de, Luis Benitez-Bribiesca. "Cytologic Detection of Vaginal Parasitosis." *Acta Cytologica.* Vol. 17, No. 3, 252-257, 1973.

Triggle, D.J. "Calcium, the Control of Smooth Muscle Function and Bronchial Hyperreactivity." *Allergy.* 38, 1-9, 1983.

Ursing, Bo, Thor Alm, Franz Barany, Ingemar Bergelin, Karin Ganrot-Norlin, Jurgen Hoevels, Bernhard Huitfeldt, Gunnar Jarnerot, Urban Krause, Aud Krook, Bjorn Lindstrom, Orjan Nordle, Anders Rosen. "A Comparative Study of Metronidazole and Sulfasalazine for Active Crohn's Disease: The Cooperative Crohn's Disease Study in Sweden. II. Result." *Gastroenterology.* 83:550-62, 1982.

Ursing, B., C. Kamme. "Metronidazole for Crohn's Disease." *The Lancet.* 775-776, Apr. 5, 1975.

Vaitukaitis, J., J.B. Robbins, E. Nieschlag, G.T. Ross. "A Method for Producing Specific Antisera with Small Doses of Immunogen." *J. Clin. Endocr.* 33:988-991, 1971.

Van Tongeren, J.H. "Rheumatoid-Factor-Like Globulins and Tropical Parasitic Infections." *The Lancet,* 1266, June 4, 1966.

Vaughan, John H. "Rheumatoid Arthritis: Evidence for a Defect in T-Cell Function." *Hospital Practice.* 101-107, May 1984.

Venkatesh, Ravindra, Soman Ninan Abraham, Isaac John, Laszlo Joseph Egler. "Recovery of Soil Amebas from the Nasal Passages of Children During the Dusty Harmattan period in Zaria." *Am. J. Clin. Path.* Vol. 71, 201-203, 1979.

Veys, E.M., Ph. Hermanns, H. Mielants, G. Verbruggen. "Mechanism of Flu-Like Syndrome Induced by Levamisole Can Be the Base of Its Mode of Action in Rheumatoid Arthritis." *Advances in Inflammation Research.* Vol. 6, 239-249, 1984.

Visvesvara, G.S., W. Balamuth. "Comparative Studies on Related Free-Living and Pathogenic Amebae with Special Reference to *Acanthamoeba.*" *Protozool.* 22(2), 245-256, 1975.

Visvesvara, G.S., Dan B. Jones, Nettie M. Robinson. "Isolation, Identification, and Biological Characterization of *Acanthamoeba Polyphaga* from a Human Eye." *The American Journal of Tropical Medicine and Hygiene,* Vol. 24, No. 5, 784-790, 1975.

Walker, J. "Relief from Chronic Pain by Low Power Laser Irradiation." *Neuroscience Letters.* 43, 339-344, 1983.

Wang, S. and Feldman, H. "Occurrence of *Acanthamoeba* in Tissue Cultures Inoculated with Human Pharyngeal Swabs." *Antimicrob. Agents Chemother.,* Vol. 1, 50-53, 1961.

_____. "Isolation of Hartmannella Species from Human Throats." *The New England Journal of Medicine,* Vol. 277, No. 22, Nov. 30, 1174-1179, 1967.

Warhurst, D. & Armstrong, J. "Study of a Small Amoeba from Mammalian Cell Cultures Infected with 'Ryan Virus'." *J. Gen. Microbiol.* Vol. 50, 207-215, 1968.

Warhurst, D., Stamm, W. & Phillips, E. "*Acanthamoeba* from a New Case of Corneal Ulcer." *Roy. Soc. Trop. Med. & Hyg. Transactions,* Vol. 70, 279, 1976.

Warthin, Aldred Scott. "The Excretion of Spirochaeta Pallida Through the Kidneys." *Arch. Opthalmol.,* 52, 525-545, 1923

_____. "The Occurrence of Entamoeba Histolytica with Tissue Lesions in the Testis and Epididymis in Chronic Dysentery." *Jour. Infect. Dis.* Vol. 30, 559-568, 1922.

Weiss, S., Kisch, E.S., Fischel, B. "Systemic Effects of Intraarticular Administration of Triamcinolone Hexacetonide," *Isr. J. Med. Sci.* Vol. 19, 83-84, 1983.

Wellings, F., Lewis, A., Amuso, P. & Chang, S. "Naegleria and Water Sports." *The Lancet.* Jan. 22, 199-200, 1977.

Wessel, Henry B., Jeffrey Hubbard, A. Julio Martinez, Eddy Willaert. "Granulomatous Amebic Encephalitis(GAE) with Prolonged Clinical Course: CT Scan Findings, Diagnosis by Brain Biopsy, and Effect of Treatment." *Neurology 30.* Vol. 30, 442, April 1980.

Wilkinson, A.E., P. Rodin, J.A. McFadzean, S. Squires. "A Note On the Effect of Metronidazole on the Nichols Strain of *Treponema pallidum in vitro* and *in vivo.*" *Brit. J. Vener. Dis.,* Vol. 43, 201-203, 1967.

Willaert, E. & Stevens, A. "Isolation of Pathogenic Amoeba from Thermal-Discharge Water." *The Lancet.,* 741, Oct. 2, 1976.

Willaert, E., Stevens, A. & Healy, G. "Retrospective identification of *Acanthamoeba culbertsoni* in a Case of Amoebic Meningoencephalitis." *Journal of Clinical Pathology,* Vol. 31, 717-720, 1978.

Wilmot, A., Powell, S. & Adams, E. "Chloroquine Compared with Chloroquine and Emetine Combined in Amebic Liver Abscess." *Am J. Trop. Med. Hyg.,* Vol. 8, 623-624, 1959.

Wilson, D., et al. "Induction of Amebiasis in Tissues of White Mice & Rats by Subcutaneous Inoculation of Small, Free-Living, Inquilinic, and Parasitic Amoebas with Associated Coliform Bacteria." *Experimental Parasitology,* Vol. 21, 277-286, 1967.

Wojtulewski, P.J., Gow, J. Walter, R. Grahame, T. Gibson, G.S. Panayi, J. Mason. "Clotrimazole in Rheumatoid Arthritis." *Annals of the Rheumatic Dis.* 39, 469-472, 1980.

_____. "Clotrimazole in Rheumatoid Arthritis." *Unpublished addenda to the above report showing effectiveness at higher levels.*) Personal Correspondence from Wojtulewski to John R.A. Simoons. 6 Pages, undated.

Wolfe, M. "Giardiasis." *J.A.M.A.* Vol. 233, No. 13, 1362-1365, 1975.

Wyburn-Mason, Roger. "The Causation of Rheumatoid Disease and Many Human Cancers." Book Report. *The Lancet.* 758, Apr. 7, 1979.

_____. "Clotrimazole and Rheumatoid Arthritis." *The Lancet.* 489, Feb. 28, 1976.

_____. "Dehydroemetine in Chronic Leukaemia." *The Lancet.* 1266-1267, June 4, 1966.

_____. "Metronidazole in Rheumatoid Arthritis." *SA Medical Journal.* 648-649, May 1, 1982.

_____. "Metronidazole in Rheumatoid Arthritis." *SA Medical Journal.* 648, (Reprint with reply by Dr. Pybus) May 1, 1982.

_____. "The Naeglerial Causation of Rheumatoid Disease and Many Human Cancers. A New Concept in Medicine." *Medical Hypotheses,* Vol. 5, 1237-1249, 1979.

Yoshikawa, Thomas, Sharon Miyamoto, Anthony W. Chow, Lucien B. Guze. "In Vitro Resistance of *Neisseria Gonorrhoeae* to Metronidazole." *Antimicrobial Agents and Chemotherapy,* Vol. 6, No. 3, 327-329, Sept. 1974.

Zaman, V. "Studies in the Immobilization Reaction in the Genus *Entamoeba.*" *Ann. Trop. Med. & Parasit.,* Vol. 54, 381-391, 1960.

135

THE RHEUMATOID DISEASE FOUNDATION
Rt. 4, Box 137, Franklin, TN 37064 **(615) 646-1030**
A non-profit, tax exempt, charitable organization

† PHYSICIAN & SCIENTIST ADVISORY LIST†

Licensed physicians below have indicated to *The Rheumatoid Disease Foundation* that they either use or are willing to use antiamoebics in the treatment of rheumatoid disease.

If the physician is starred (*), then he/she is also willing to use the Wyburn-Mason/Pybus/Bourne intraneural injection technique for the pain resulting from RD damage and/or the treatment of osteoarthritis.

The Rheumatoid Disease Foundation provides this list as a public service to those who inquire. Inclusion of physicians in this referral list does not indicate an endorsement of any physician's practice nor a guarantee of effectiveness of treatment.

If your family physician inquires of *The Rheumatoid Disease Foundation*, he/she will be referred to one of the Advisory Member physicians or scientists and will be provided with a protocol for your treatment.

The Rheumatoid Disease Foundation assumes no financial obligation for the service of physician referral.

Important Note
We recommend that you first go to your family doctor. If he refuses to treat you, then try the physicians in this list. Since new physicians are joining each week, you may also wish to write to *The Rheumatoid Disease Foundation* for the latest list.

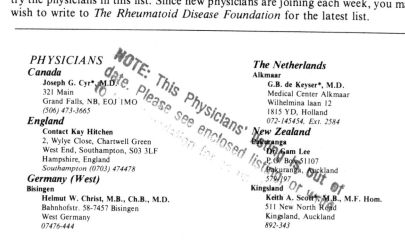

PHYSICIANS

Canada
Joseph G. Cyr*, M.D.
321 Main
Grand Falls, NB, EOJ 1MO
(506) 473-3665

England
Contact Kay Hitchen
2, Wylie Close, Chartwell Green
West End, Southampton, S03 3LF
Hampshire, England
Southampton (0703) 474478

Germany (West)
Bisingen
Helmut W. Christ, M.B., Ch.B., M.D.
Bahnhofstr. 58-7457 Bisingen
West Germany
07476-444

The Netherlands
Alkmaar
G.B. de Keyser*, M.D.
Medical Center Alkmaar
Wilhelmina laan 12
1815 YD, Holland
072-145454, Ext. 2584

New Zealand
Pakuranga
Dr. Gam Lee
P.O. Box 51107
Pakuranga, Auckland
579/197

Kingsland
Keith A. Scott*, M.B., M.F. Hom.
511 New North Road
Kingsland, Auckland
892-343

Puerto Rico

Guillermo Ulmos*, M.D.
Calle Espinosa 373
Borinquen Gardens
Rio Piedras, Puerto Rico 00828
Phone number unknown

Republic of Korea (South)

Jeoung Pyung Eup
Anna M. Boland, M.M., M.D.
Maryknoll Sisters Clinic
Jeoung Pyung Eup, Chung Pukto
South Korea (ROK) N311
Phone Unknown

Republic of South Africa

Contact Paul Pybus
404 United Bldg, 181 Church Street
Natal, Pietermaritzburg 3201
27-331-57675

United States

Alabama
H. Ray Evers*, M.D.
600 Mineral Wells Road
P.O. Box 587
Cottonwood, AL 36320
(205) 691-2161
James M. Foster, M.D.
600 Mineral Wells Road
P.O. Box 587
Cottonwood, AL 36320
(205) 691-2161
Samuel Fischer III, M.D.
1016 18th St. South
Birmingham, AL 35205
(205) 933-1958
Pat Hamm*, M.D.
3804 6th Ave. W.
Huntsville, AL 35805
(205) 534-8115
John Kerr, M.D.
Hamilton, AL 35570
(205) 921-3153
Gus J. Prosch*, Jr., M.D.
244 Goodwin Crest Drive
Suite 312
Birmingham, AL 35209
(205) 942-8985
Arizona
Lloyd D. Armold, D.O.
2525 S. Rural Rd., Suite 4
Tempe, AZ 85282
(602) 967-7557
Abram Ber, M.D.
3134 N. 7th St.
Phoenix, AZ 85014
(602) 279-3795
H.C. Purtzer, D.O.
13825 N. 7th St., Suite H
Phoenix, AZ 85022
(602) 942-6944
Francis J. Woo, Jr., M.D.
60 Riviera Drive
Lake Havasu City, AZ 86403
(602) 453-3330
Arkansas
Wayne Smith, M.D.
Family Clinic
P.O. Box 569
Hardy, AR 72542
(501) 856-3213
Charles Swingle, M.D.
105 Nathan
Marked Tree, AR 72365
(501) 358-2036

California
Laszlo I. Belenyessy*, M.D.
Yale-Wilshire Medical Building
2901 Wilshire Blvd., Suite 435
Santa Monica, CA 90403
(213) 828-4480
Robert Bingham*, M.D.
Desert Arthritis Medical Clinic
13-630 Mountain View Road
Desert Hot Springs, CA 92240
(619) 329-6422
7750 Katella Ave.
Stanton, CA 90680
(714) 891-4443
William C. Bryce, M.D.
17220 Newhope St., Suite 109
Fountain Valley, CA 92708
(714) 557-3867
Orville J. Davis, M.D.
4224 Ohio Street
San Diego, CA 92104
(619) 283-6033
David J. Edwards*, M.D.
6154 N. Amber
Fresno, CA 93727
(209) 251-5066
Robert B. Gold*, D.O.
1905 N. College Ave., Suite B2
Santa Ana, CA 92706
(707) 541-4080
Robert L. Harmon, M.D.
43-576 Washington St.
Palm Desert, CA 92260
(619) 345-2696
H.J. Hoegerman*, MD
101 W. Arrellaga
Santa Barbara, CA 93101
(805) 963-1624
M. Jahangiri*, M.D.
2156 Santa Fe Ave.
Los Angeles, CA 90058
(213) 587-3218
Eva Jalkotzy*, M.D.
1560 Hartnell Ave.
Redding, CA 96002
(916) 222-0116
Zane Kime, M.D.
1212 High St., Suite 204
Auburn, CA 95603
(916) 823-3421
Richard A. Kunin, M.D.
2698 Pacific Ave.
San Francisco, CA 94115
(415) 346-2500
A.H. Kryger, M.D.
Nutrition — Preventive Medicine
P.O. Box 1927
Lincoln Near Eighth
Carmel by the Sea, CA 93921
(408) 624-4663
Carl V. Lansing*, M.D
Crescent City, CA 95531
(707) 464-2144
Emil Levin, M.D.
8540 South Sepulveda Blvd
Suite 910
Los Angeles, CA 90045
(213) 776-5123
Paul Lynn , M.D.
345 W. Portal
San Francisco, CA 94127
(415) 566-1000

Glen C. Mahoney, M.D.
Health Resource Center
7442 Mountjoy Drive
Huntington Beach, CA 92648
(714) 841-2803
Emmanuel Mojtahedian*, M.D.
6425 Whittier Blvd.
Los Angeles, CA 90022
(213) 728-0101
Frank J. Mosler*, M.D.
14428 Gilmore St.
Van Nuys, CA 91401
(818) 785-7425
James R. Privitera, M.D.
105 North Grandview Ave.
Covina, CA 91723
(818) 966-1618
William J. Saccoman, M.D.
505 N. Mollison, N103
El Cajon, CA 92021
(619) 440-3838
Elden B. Shields*, M.D.
407-A Potter Street
Fallbrook, CA 92028
(714) 728-1147

Colorado
William Doell, D.O.
4045 Wadsworth Blvd.
Wheatridge, CO 80033
(303) 422-0585
Hugh Kragor*, D.O.
North Lowell Medical Clinic
7325 Lowell Blvd.
Westminster, CO 80030
(303) 428-7571

District of Columbia
(Washington, D.C.)
H.E. Sartori*, M.D.
4501 Connecticut Ave NW, No. 306
Washington, D.C. 20008
(202) 244-6215
(202) 244-6327

Florida
Ervin Barr*, D.O.
Family Medicine
2350 W. Oakland Park Blvd.
Ft. Lauderdale, FL 33311
(305) 731-8080
Donald J. Carrow*, M.D.
The Largo Center for
  Preventive & General Medicine
1501 S. Belcher Rd.
Largo, FL 33541
(813) 536-3531
Martin Dayton*,D.O.
18600 Collins Ave.
Miami, FL 33160
(305) 931-8484
J. Gordon Godorov*, D.O.
9055 SW 87th Ave., Suite 307
Miami, FL 33176
(305) 595-0671
George F. Graves, D.O.
Fort McCoy Medical Center
PO Box P
Ft. McCoy, FL 32637
(904) 236-2525
W.W. Mittelstadt*, M.D./D.O.
1736 East Commercial Blvd.
Fort Lauderdale, FL 33334
(305) 772-4838
Alfred S. Massam*, MD
PO Box 1328
Wauchula, FL 33873
(813) 773-6668

John P. McVay*, D.O.
The Largo Center for
  Preventive and General Medicine
1501 S. Belcher
Largo, FL 33541
(813) 536-3531
W.R. Rundles*, M.D.
Sweet Water Medical-Surgical Clinic
5795 Taylor Branch Rd
Port Orange, FL 32019
(904) 756-0064
Richard J. Sabates, M.D.
1758 E. Commercial Blvd.
Ft. Lauderdale, FL 33334
(305) 771-1220
Myron Timken*, D.O.
2280 U.S. Hwy 19 N
Suite 265-D
Clearwater, FL 33575
(813) 796-1831

Georgia
William C. Douglass*, M.D.
The Douglass Center
2550 Windy Hill Rd, Suite 315
Marietta, GA 30067
(404) 953-0710

Hawaii
R. H. Renn, D.O.
1909 Ala Wai Blvd. N1602
Honolulu, HI 96815
(808) 942-2000

Illinois
Leonard J. Braudo, M.D.
Fahey Medical Center
581 Golf Rd.
Des Plaines, IL 60016
(312) 297-2240
M.P. Dommers, M.D.
554 South Main
Belvidere, IL 61008
(815) 544-3112
T. Hesselink, M.D.
554 South Main
Belvidere, IL 61008
(815) 544-3112
William F.P. Phillips*, M.D.
5307 Devon Avenue
Chicago, IL 60646
(312) 774-1725
Ralph H. Roeper*, D.O.
121 N. Northwest Hwy.
Palatine, IL 60067
(312) 358-2257
John R. Tambone*, M.D.
102 E. South Street
Woodstock, IL 60098
(815) 338-2345
Robert S. Waters, M.D.
Waters Preventive Medical Center, Inc.
1435 S. Roselle Rd.
Schaumburg, IL 60172
(312) 894-1790

Indiana
David Darbro, M.D.
Darbro Foundation
  for Medical Preventics, Inc.
2124 E. Hanna Ave.
Indianapolis, IN 46227
(317) 787-7221
Cal Streeter, D.O.
3313-45th Street
Highland, IN 46322
(219) 924-2410
202 Main Street
Middlebury, IN 46540
(219) 825-9618

138

David E. Turfler, D.O.
336 West Navarre St.
South Bend, IN 46616
(219) 233-3840
Norman Whitney, D.O.
P.O. Box 173
Mooresville, IN 46158
(317) 831-3352
Kentucky
Kirk D. Morgan*, M.D.
9501 U.S. 42
Prospect, KY 40059
(502) 228-0156
3101 Breckenridge Lane
Louisville, KY 40220
(502) 459-0315
Louisiana
Roy M. Montalbano*, M.D.
1323 S. Tyler St., Suite 105
Covington, LA 70433
(504) 893-5683
Massachusetts
Michael Janson, M.D.
2557 Massachusetts Ave.
Cambridge, MA 02140
(617) 661-6225
Maine
Joseph G. Cyr*, M.D.
62 Main St.
Van Buren, ME 04785
(207) 868-5273
Maryland
Paul V. Beals, M.D.
9101 Cherry Lane Park
Laurel, MD 20708
(301) 490-9911
Alan Gaby, M.D.
19 Walker Ave.
Pikesville, MD 21208
(301) 486-5656
Michigan
Vahagn Agbabian*, D.O.
Pontiac State Bank Bldg. N1105
28 N. Saginaw Street
Pontiac, MI 48058
(313) 334-2424
Seldon Nelson*, D.O.
Williamston Medical Bldg.
1435 E. Grand River Ave.
Williamston, MI 48895
(517) 655-4381
Richard L. Plagenhoef, M.D.
1849 R.W. Berends Dr., S.W.
Wyoming, MI 49509
(616) 358-6461
207 South North St.
Otsego, MI 49078
(616) 694-9496
Earle J. Reynolds, D.O.
Standale Medical Center,P.C.
3950 Lake Michigan Drive NW
Grand Rapids, MI 49504
(616) 453-2429
Harley J. Robinson*, D.O.
20101 Greenfield
Detroit, MI 48235
(313) 273-1510, 273-1511
Richard E. Tapert, D.O.
15850 E. Warren
Detroit, MI 48224
(313) 885-5405
H. William Winstanley, D.O.
Clawson Urgent Care Center
625 West Fourteen Mile Rd.
Clawson, MI 48017
(313) 435-8630

Mississippi
Jack M. Blount, M.D.
580 East Main Street
Philadelphia, MS 39350
(601) 656-3811
R. T. Hollingsworth*, M.D.
Hollingsworth Shelby Clinic, Ltd.
Drawer 87
Shelby, MS 38774
(601) 398-5106
Missouri
Bob R. Carnett*, D.O.
Salem Medical Clinic
Rolla Rd at McArthur St.
Salem, MO 65560
(314) 729-7311
Martin H. Christ, M.D.
1402 Faraon St.
St. Joseph, MO 64501
(816) 279-1615
James L. Rowland*, D.O.
8133 Wornall Rd
Kansas City, MO 64114
(816) 361-4077
L.A. Weisman*, D.O.
Shell Knob Medical Center
Shell Knob, MO 65747
(417) 858-3131
New Jersey
M.J. Packovich, M.D.
228 Route 17 North
Upper Saddle River, NJ 07458
(201) 825-8810
Marvin H. Soalt*, D.O.
110A Troy Towers
PO Box 1429
Bloomfield, NJ 07003
(201) 743-2716
New Mexico
E.L. Miller, D.O.
401 South Avenue A
Portales, NM 88130
(505) 356-4471
New York
Mitchell Kurk, M.D.
310 Broadway
Lawrence, NY 11559
(516) 239-5540
Warren M. Levin, M.D.
World Health Medical Group
444 Park Ave. South (at 30th St.)
New York, NY 10016
(212) 696-1900
Michael B. Schachter, M.D.
Mountainview Medical Building
Mountainview Avenue
Nyack, NY 10960
(914) 358-6800
Harold Weiss, M.D.
8002 19th Avenue
Brooklyn, NY 11214
(212) 236-2202
North Carolina
John L. Laird, M.D.
Great Smokies Medical Center
Rt. 1, Box 7
Leicester, NC 28748
(704) 683-3101
Logan T. Robertson, M.D.
Route 2
Canton, NC 28716
(704) 235-9112
Ted Rozema, M.D.
4505 Fair Meadows Lane
Raleigh, NC 27607
(919) 781-8686

Paul Sale, M.D.
P.O. Drawer 640
Bryson City, NC 28713
(704) 488-2162
Philip M. Toyama*, M.D.
Friendship Center Office Park
Suite 600
Greensboro, NC 27409
(919) 292-7025
North Dakota
Brian E. Briggs, M.D.
718 Sixth St. SW
Minot, North Dakota 58701
(701) 838-6011
Ohio
J.M. Baron*, D.O.
3101 Euclid Ave., Suite 201
Cleveland, OH 44115
(216) 432-2277
Heather Morgan, M.D.
Self-Health Institutes
138 South Main Street
Centerville, OH 45459
(513) 439-1797
Harold J. Wilson, M.D.
28 W. Henderson Rd.
Columbus, OH 43214
(614) 261-0151
If no answer: (614) 299-4151
Oklahoma
Charles H. Farr*, M.D.
1312 NW 12th St.
Suite 108
Moore, OK 73170
(405) 799-8781
P.R. Riemer*, D.O.
Hillcrest Medical Center
700 Denver
Pawnee, OK 74058
(918) 762-2542
Oregon
John E. Gambee, M.D.
66 Club Rd., Suite 140
Eugene, OR 97401
(503) 686-2536
Pennsylvania
Harold Buttram, M.D.
Clymer Medical Building
RD N3, Clymer Road
Quakertown, PA 18951
(215) 536-1890
P. Jayalakshmi*, M.D.
New Life Center
6366 Sherwood Rd.
Philadelphia, PA 19151
(215) 473-4226, 473-7453
Donald J. Mantell, M.D.
RD 1, Box 286
Old Mars-Criders Road
Evans City, PA 16033
(412) 776-5610
M.J. Packovich, M.D.
215 Crooked Run Rd.
North Versailles, PA 15137
(412) 673-3900
Ronald M. Repice, M.D.
1502 Upland Street
Chester, PA 19013
(215) 874-1500
K.R. Sampathachar*, M.D.
New Life Center
6366 Sherwood Rd.
Philadelphia, PA 19151
(215) 473-4226, 473-7453

Eugene R. Shippen, M.D.
7 East Lancaster Avenue
Shillington, PA 19607
(215) 777-7896
Theodore B. Tihansky, M.D.
Medical Arts Building
Schuykill Haven, PA 17972
(717) 385-1578
Harold C. Walmer*, D.O.
50 North Market St.
Elizabethtown, PA 17022
(717) 367-1345
South Carolina
Robert M. Johnson*, M.D.
7499 Northforest Drive
Charleston, SC 29405
(803) 797-7033
Ted Rozema, M.D.
1000 E. Rutherford Rd
Landrum, SC 29356
(803) 457-4141
William F. Ward, Jr., M.D.
Total Health Center
1720 Augusta Rd
West Columbia, SC 29169
(803) 791-4615
South Dakota
L.L. Therberge*, D.O.
814 Columbus St.
Rapid City, SD 57701
(605) 342-0523
Tennessee
Stuart P. Bacon, M.D.
Rhea Family Physicians, P.C.
Rhea County Professional Building
1912 Hwy. 27 North
Dayton, TN 37231
(615) 775-4261
M.R. Caldwell, D.O.
Soddy Daisy, TN 37379
(615) 332-1578
Archimedes A. Concon, M.D.
4939 Princeton Road
Memphis, TN 38117
(901) 323-5808
Fred M. Furr, M.D.
9217 Park West Blvd.
Building E, Suite 1
Knoxville, TN 37923
(615) 683-1502
Fulton J. Greer*, M.D.
Confederate Medical Building
Carters Creek Pike
Franklin, TN 37064
(615) 794-8431
7028 Church St. E.
Brentwood, TN 37027
(615) 373-4330
Donald C. Thompson, M.D.
1121 W. 1st No. St.
Morristown, TN 37814
(615) 581-6367
Eugene S. Wolcott* M.D.
495 Centennial
Lewisburg, TN 37091
(615) 359-1533
Texas
Jim P. Archer*, D.O.
Weber Road Clinic
5202 Weber Road
Corpus Christi, TX 78411
(512) 852-4031

140

Robert M. Battle, M.D.
140 South Parking Place
Lake Jackson, TX 77566
(409) 297-6434
Daniel E. Bruhl, M.D.
3815 Fannin
Houston, TX 77004
(713) 522-7605
Joseph F. Carbone*, D.O.
Coastal Bend Medical Center
1501 E. Red River
Victoria, TX 77901
(512) 575-6665
Stevan Cordas, D.O.
1100 W. Airport Freeway
(Near DFW Airport)
Bedford, TX 76022
(817) 267-8181
R.M. Davis*, M. D.
2032 Hialeah
Seabrook, TX 77586
(713) 474-3236
William W. Halcomb*, D.O.
8311 Shoal Creek Blvd.
Austin, TX 78758
(512) 451-8149
G. Juetersonke, D.O.
1501 Merrimac Circle
Ft. Worth, TX 76107
(817) 870-5230
A. L. Karbach, D.O.
314 North Center
Arlington, TX 76011
(817) 274-8417
Gerald M. Parker, D.O.
4714 S. Western
Amarillo, TX 79109
(806) 355-8203
John L. Sessions*, D.O.
Jasper County Medical Center
1609 South Margaret
Kirbyville, TX 75956
(409) 423-2166
Eva Lee Snead, M.D.
Family Practice and Nutrition
437 W. Magnolia
San Antonio, TX 78212
(512) 736-5643
Jack K. Taylor, D.O.
3749 39th Street
Port Arthur, TX 77642
(409) 982-1391
John Parks Trowbridge*, M.D.
9816 Memorial, Suite 205
Humble, TX 77338
(713) 540-2329
Robert B. Vance*, D.O.
9910 Long Point Road
Houston, TX 77055
(713) 932-0552
Jack R. Vinson, D.O.
Preventive Medicine Center
4315 Alpha Road
Dallas, TX 75234
(214) 239-8844
Robert T. Warhola*, D.O.
1100 NASA Rd. 1
Suite 300
Houston, TX 77058
(713) 486-0660
Donald R. Whitaker*, D.O.
1800 Judson Road
Longview, TX 75601
(214) 758-3989

Utah
Cordell E. Logan, N.M.D.
1773 West 7000 South
West Jordan, UT 84084
(801) 562-2211
West Virginia
Albert V. Jellen, M.D.
2097 National Road
Wheeling, WV 26003
(304) 242-5151
Washington
Murray L. Black, D.O.
622 S. 36th Ave.
Yakima, WA 98902
(509) 966-1780
David Buscher, M.D.
121 3rd Ave.
Kirkland, WA 98033
(206) 827-2151
Quentin G. Schwenke, M.D.
321 Wellington St.
Walla Walla, WA 99362
(509) 525-4070

SCIENTISTS
Arizona
William E. Catterall, Sc.D.
(Nutritionist)
5929 East 32nd St.
Tucson, AZ 85711
(602) 790-2684
North Carolina
John R.A. Simoons, Ph.D.
(Pharmacologist)
5140 Revere Road
Parkwood
Durham, NC 27713
(919) 544-4040
Oklahoma
Dr. Jon Tillinghast
13516 Pecan
Edmond, OK 73034
(405) 755-2720
Tennessee
Frederick H. Binford, B.S., M.A.
(Physicist)
1803 Morena Street
Nashville, TN 37208
(615) 329-0823:H (615) 329-8623:O
Vermont
Dr J. Rinse
East Dorset, VT 05253
(802) 362-3306

141

HELP SPREAD THE Good NEWS !

Do you have a friend, neighbor or loved one who is suffering—perhaps needlessly—from the constant pain of arthritis? Just fill out the back of this form, and we'll do everything we can to help.

MEMBERSHIP ENROLLMENT FORM

☐ It's time we ended the myth that there's no cure for arthritis. Please enroll me as a member of the Foundation and send me everything necessary to help spread the good news! *I have enclosed my contribution of at least $25.*

☐ In addition to my membership contribution, I have also enclosed a donation of $ _____ .

☐ I can't afford to send $25 to become a member, but I still want to help. Enclosed is my contribution of $ _____ . Please put it to good use in your efforts.

Please make check payable to: Rheumatoid Disease Foundation

Name _____

Address _____

City _____ State _____ Zip _____

Your contribution is fully tax-deductible.

DETACH AND RETURN THIS PORTION

THE
RHEUMATOID DISEASE FOUNDATION / P.O. BOX 17405, WASHINGTON, D.C. 20041

MEMBERSHIP BENEFITS

**FOR YOUR
TAX RECORDS**

Date _____

Check No. _____

Amount _____

Thank you!

Rheumatoid Disease Foundation members will receive:

- A pin showing the Foundation's symbol—the Limax amoeba;
- An automobile window decal;
- The Foundation's newsletter;
- Invitations to regional seminars;
- Printed abstracts from those seminars;
- Updates of the Physician's List;
- A Member Copy of *Rheumatoid Diseases Cured at Last.*

ALL CONTRIBUTIONS ARE TAX-DEDUCTIBLE

Please send information about the Rheumatoid Disease Foundation and its efforts to eliminate the misery and pain of rheumatoid arthritis to the names and addresses *printed* below:

Name _____

Address _____

City_____ State_____ Zip_____

Name _____

Address _____

City_____ State_____ Zip_____

Name _____

Address _____

City_____ State_____ Zip_____

Name _____

Address _____

City_____ State_____ Zip_____

Use this order blank

I am enclosing _____ for _____ copies of Anthony di Fabio's book, *Rheumatoid Diseases Cured at Last!* ($9.95 per book, plus $1.00 postage and handling). Please mail the book(s) to:

Name _____

Address _____

City _____

State _____ Zip Code _____

Mail check or money order to: The Rheumatoid Disease Foundation

Rt. 4, Box 137
Franklin, TN 37064
(615) 646-1030

THE RHEUMATOID DISEASE FOUNDATION

P.O. BOX 17405, WASHINGTON, D.C. 20041

☐ **YES,** Dr. Blount, I agree that it's time to bring the pain and suffering of 31,000,000 arthritis victims to an end.

To help you raise the funds needed to expedite the research necessary for FDA acceptance of your findings, I am enclosing my contribution of:

PLEASE CHECK ONE:

☐ $100   ☐ $75   ☐ $50   ☐ $25

☐ $15   ☐ $10   ☐ Other $ _____

Please make check payable to: Rheumatoid Disease Foundation

Name _____

Address _____

City _____

State _____ **Zip** _____

☐ **YES,** I have enclosed a contribution of $15 or more. Please rush my complimentary copy of *Rheumatoid Diseases Cured at Last.*

☐ Please check this box if you wish to receive additional copies of this authoritative book (a minimum contribution of $15 required for each copy requested).

☐ **YES,** please send me your list of reputable physicians who are employing the Foundation's effective treatment for arthritis.

THANK YOU. ALL CONTRIBUTIONS ARE TAX-DEDUCTIBLE

THE RHEUMATOID DISEASE FOUNDATION IS A PROJECT OF
THE ROGER WYBURN—MASON & JACK M. BLOUNT FOUNDATION
FOR THE ERADICATION OF RHEUMATOID DISEASE

Cut Here

Cut Here

Cut Here